2. Quinoa Salad with Roasted Vegetables

Ingredients:
- 1 cup uncooked quinoa, rinsed
- 2 cups vegetable or chicken broth
- 1 red bell pepper, chopped
- 1 zucchini, chopped
- 1 red onion, chopped
- 2 cups broccoli florets
- 2 tbsp olive oil
- 1 tsp ground cumin
- 1 tsp paprika
- 1/2 tsp salt
- 1/4 tsp black pepper
- 2 tbsp fresh lemon juice
- 2 tbsp chopped fresh parsley
- 2 tbsp chopped fresh basil

Instructions:

1. Preheat oven to 400°F. Toss the chopped bell pepper, zucchini, onion, and broccoli with the olive oil, cumin, paprika, salt, and pepper on a large baking sheet. Roast for 20-25 minutes, stirring halfway, until vegetables are tender and lightly browned.

2. Meanwhile, in a medium saucepan, combine the quinoa and broth. Bring to a boil, then reduce heat to low, cover and simmer for 15-20 minutes until quinoa is tender and liquid is absorbed. Fluff with a fork.

3. In a large bowl, combine the roasted vegetables and cooked quinoa. Stir in the lemon juice, parsley, and basil.

4. Serve the quinoa salad warm or chilled. Enjoy!

This salad is packed with anti-inflammatory ingredients like quinoa, vegetables, and fresh herbs. The roasted veggies add great flavor and texture. It's a delicious and nutritious option for those dealing with arthritis or inflammation.

3. Vegetable Stir-Fry with Tofu

Ingredients:
- 1 block (14 oz) extra-firm tofu, drained and cubed
- 2 tbsp sesame oil, divided
- 2 cloves garlic, minced
- 1 tbsp grated fresh ginger
- 1 red bell pepper, sliced
- 1 cup broccoli florets
- 1 cup sliced mushrooms
- 1 cup snow peas or snap peas
- 2 green onions, sliced
- 2 tbsp low-sodium soy sauce
- 1 tbsp rice vinegar
- 1 tsp sesame seeds (optional)

Instructions:

1. In a large skillet or wok, heat 1 tbsp of the sesame oil over medium-high heat. Add the cubed tofu and cook, stirring occasionally, until lightly browned on all sides, about 5-7 minutes. Transfer the tofu to a plate.

2. In the same skillet, heat the remaining 1 tbsp sesame oil over medium-high heat. Add the garlic and ginger and cook for 1 minute, stirring constantly, until fragrant.

3. Add the bell pepper, broccoli, mushrooms, and snow peas. Stir-fry for 4-5 minutes, until the vegetables are tender-crisp.

4. Return the cooked tofu to the skillet. Add the soy sauce and rice vinegar. Toss everything together and cook for 2-3 minutes more, until heated through.

5. Remove from heat and stir in the sliced green onions.

6. Serve the vegetable stir-fry immediately, garnished with sesame seeds if desired. Enjoy!

This stir-fry is packed with a variety of fresh vegetables and protein-rich tofu. The ginger, garlic, and soy sauce provide great Asian-inspired flavor. It's a healthy, delicious, and easy-to-make vegetarian dish.

Welcome to ***"Healing Recipes and Anti-Inflammatory Tips",*** your comprehensive guide to managing arthritis through the power of food. Whether you've recently been diagnosed with arthritis or have been living with it for years, this book aims to provide you with delicious, easy-to-make recipes and practical tips to help reduce inflammation and improve your quality of life.

Arthritis, a condition characterized by inflammation of the joints, affects millions of people worldwide. The pain, stiffness, and swelling associated with arthritis can significantly impact daily activities and overall well-being. While medication and other treatments play a crucial role in managing arthritis, recent research has highlighted the importance of diet in reducing inflammation and supporting joint health.

This book is designed to be your culinary companion on the journey to better health. Inside, you will find a collection of recipes that prioritize anti-inflammatory ingredients known for their healing properties. From vibrant salads packed with fresh vegetables and healthy fats to hearty main courses rich in lean proteins and whole grains, every recipe is crafted to nourish your body and delight your taste buds.

In addition to the recipes, we've included valuable tips and insights into the role of nutrition in managing arthritis. You'll learn about specific foods that can help reduce inflammation, the importance of maintaining a balanced diet, and practical strategies for incorporating these foods into your daily meals. We also provide guidance on meal planning, shopping for arthritis-friendly ingredients, and cooking techniques that preserve the nutritional integrity of your food.

We understand that living with arthritis can be challenging, and making dietary changes might seem daunting at first. However, our goal is to make this transition as enjoyable and straightforward as possible. The recipes in this book are designed to be simple yet flavorful, requiring minimal preparation time so that you can focus on enjoying your meals without added stress.

Whether you are an experienced home cook or a kitchen novice, ***"Healing Recipes and Anti-Inflammatory Tips"*** offers something for everyone. We hope that this book not only helps you manage your arthritis symptoms but also brings joy and satisfaction to your dining experience.

Thank you for choosing this book as your guide to a healthier, more comfortable life. Let's embark on this culinary journey together and discover the healing power of food.

Warm regards,

1. Grilled Salmon with Lemon and Dill

Ingredients:
- 4 salmon fillets (about 6 oz each)
- 2 tbsp olive oil
- 2 tbsp fresh lemon juice
- 2 tsp chopped fresh dill
- 1 tsp grated lemon zest
- 1/2 tsp salt
- 1/4 tsp black pepper

Instructions:

1. Preheat grill to medium-high heat.

2. In a small bowl, whisk together the olive oil, lemon juice, dill, lemon zest, salt, and pepper.

3. Place the salmon fillets on a plate and brush the top side with the lemon-dill mixture.

4. Grill the salmon for 4-6 minutes per side, or until it flakes easily with a fork. Baste the salmon with any remaining lemon-dill mixture during the last minute of cooking.

5. Serve the grilled salmon immediately, garnished with extra fresh dill if desired. Enjoy!

The bright lemon and fragrant dill pair beautifully with the rich salmon for a delicious and healthy grilled fish dish.

4. Lentil Soup with Spinach

Ingredients:
- 1 tbsp olive oil
- 1 onion, diced
- 3 cloves garlic, minced
- 1 cup brown or green lentils, rinsed
- 6 cups low-sodium vegetable or chicken broth
- 1 (14.5 oz) can diced tomatoes
- 1 tsp ground cumin
- 1 tsp dried oregano
- 1/2 tsp smoked paprika
- 1/4 tsp red pepper flakes (optional)
- Salt and black pepper to taste
- 4 cups fresh spinach, chopped

Instructions:
1. In a large pot or Dutch oven, heat the olive oil over medium heat. Add the diced onion and sauté for 5 minutes until translucent.

2. Add the minced garlic and sauté for 1 minute more, until fragrant.

3. Stir in the rinsed lentils, broth, diced tomatoes, cumin, oregano, smoked paprika, and red pepper flakes (if using). Season with salt and pepper to taste.

4. Bring the soup to a boil, then reduce heat and let simmer for 20-25 minutes, until the lentils are tender.

5. Stir in the chopped fresh spinach and cook for 2-3 minutes more, until the spinach is wilted.

6. Taste and adjust seasonings as needed.

7. Serve the lentil soup hot, garnished with extra black pepper, a squeeze of lemon, or a sprinkle of Parmesan cheese if desired.

This lentil soup is hearty, nutritious, and full of flavor from the spices and fresh spinach. Lentils are a great source of plant-based protein, fiber, and minerals. It's a comforting and satisfying soup that's perfect for a chilly day.

5. Spinach and Strawberry Salad with Walnuts

Ingredients:
- 5 oz baby spinach leaves
- 1 cup fresh strawberries, sliced
- 1/4 cup chopped walnuts
- 2 tbsp crumbled feta cheese (optional)
- 2 tbsp balsamic vinegar
- 1 tbsp olive oil
- 1 tsp Dijon mustard
- 1 tsp honey
- Salt and pepper to taste

Instructions:

1. In a large salad bowl, combine the baby spinach leaves, sliced strawberries, chopped walnuts, and crumbled feta cheese (if using).

2. In a small bowl, whisk together the balsamic vinegar, olive oil, Dijon mustard, and honey until well combined. Season with a pinch of salt and pepper.

3. Drizzle the balsamic vinaigrette over the salad and toss gently to coat.

4. Serve the spinach and strawberry salad immediately.

Optional Variations:
- Add grilled chicken or shrimp for a heartier main dish salad.

- Swap the feta for goat cheese or blue cheese.

- Use toasted pecans or almonds instead of walnuts.

- Add a sprinkle of poppy seeds or chia seeds.

This salad is a delicious and nutritious combination of fresh spinach, sweet strawberries, crunchy walnuts, and a tangy balsamic vinaigrette. The flavors and textures complement each other perfectly. It's a great option for a light lunch or side salad.

6. Baked Chicken with Herbs

Ingredients:
- 4 boneless, skinless chicken breasts
- 2 tbsp olive oil
- 2 tsp dried thyme
- 2 tsp dried rosemary
- 1 tsp garlic powder
- 1 tsp onion powder
- 1 tsp salt
- 1/2 tsp black pepper

Instructions:

1. Preheat your oven to 400°F (200°C).

2. Pat the chicken breasts dry with paper towels and place them in a baking dish or on a rimmed baking sheet.

3. In a small bowl, combine the olive oil, dried thyme, dried rosemary, garlic powder, onion powder, salt, and black pepper. Mix well to create a herb seasoning mixture.

4. Rub the herb seasoning mixture all over the chicken breasts, making sure to coat them evenly on both sides.

5. Bake the chicken in the preheated oven for 25-30 minutes, or until the internal temperature reaches 165°F (75°C) when measured with a meat thermometer.

6. Remove the baked chicken from the oven and let it rest for 5 minutes before serving.

Serving Suggestions:
- Serve the baked chicken with roasted vegetables, mashed potatoes, or a fresh salad.
- Garnish the chicken with fresh chopped parsley or thyme for extra flavor.
- For a creamier dish, you can make a simple pan sauce by deglazing the baking dish with a bit of chicken broth or white wine.

This baked chicken recipe is easy to prepare and packed with flavor from the aromatic herbs and spices. The chicken comes out juicy and tender every time. It's a great weeknight dinner option that the whole family will enjoy.

7. Roasted Vegetable Medley

Ingredients:
- 1 medium zucchini, cut into 1-inch pieces
- 1 medium yellow squash, cut into 1-inch pieces
- 1 red bell pepper, cut into 1-inch pieces
- 1 yellow onion, cut into 1-inch pieces
- 8 oz cremini or button mushrooms, halved
- 2 carrots, peeled and cut into 1-inch pieces
- 3 cloves garlic, minced
- 2 tbsp olive oil
- 1 tsp dried thyme
- 1 tsp dried oregano
- 1/2 tsp salt
- 1/4 tsp black pepper

Instructions:
1. Preheat your oven to 400°F (200°C). Line a large baking sheet with parchment paper or foil.

2. In a large bowl, combine the chopped zucchini, yellow squash, bell pepper, onion, mushrooms, and carrots.

3. Add the minced garlic, olive oil, dried thyme, dried oregano, salt, and black pepper. Toss everything together until the vegetables are evenly coated.

4. Spread the seasoned vegetables in a single layer on the prepared baking sheet.

5. Roast the vegetables in the preheated oven for 25-30 minutes, stirring halfway, until they are tender and lightly browned. Remove the roasted vegetable medley from the oven and serve hot.

Serving Suggestions:
- Serve the roasted vegetables as a side dish, or toss them with cooked pasta or quinoa for a main course.
- Top the roasted veggies with crumbled feta or shredded parmesan cheese.
- Add a drizzle of balsamic glaze or a squeeze of lemon juice for extra flavor.
- Sprinkle with fresh chopped herbs like parsley, basil, or oregano.

This roasted vegetable medley is a simple and versatile dish that showcases a variety of colorful, nutrient-dense vegetables. The high-heat roasting brings out the natural sweetness and caramelizes the edges for a delicious, tender result.

8. Turmeric Chicken Curry

Ingredients:
- 1/2 tsp cayenne pepper (or to taste)
- 1 cup low-sodium chicken broth
- 1 (13.5 oz) can coconut milk
- 1 tsp salt
- 1/4 tsp black pepper
- 3 cloves garlic, minced
- 2 cups cooked basmati rice, for serving
- Chopped cilantro for garnish
- 1 lb boneless, skinless chicken thighs, cut into 1-inch pieces
- 2 tbsp olive oil
- 1 onion, diced
- 1 tbsp grated fresh ginger
- 2 tsp ground turmeric
- 1 tsp ground cumin
- 1 tsp ground coriander

Instructions:

1. In a large skillet or Dutch oven, heat the olive oil over medium-high heat. Add the diced onion and sauté for 3-4 minutes until translucent.

2. Add the minced garlic and grated ginger. Cook for 1 minute, stirring constantly, until fragrant.

3. Stir in the ground turmeric, cumin, coriander, and cayenne pepper. Cook for 1 minute to toast the spices.

4. Add the chicken pieces and toss to coat in the spices. Cook for 3-4 minutes, until the chicken is lightly browned.

5. Pour in the chicken broth and coconut milk. Season with salt and pepper.

6. Bring the curry to a simmer, then reduce heat to medium-low. Let the curry simmer for 15-20 minutes, until the chicken is cooked through and the sauce has thickened.

7. Serve the turmeric chicken curry over cooked basmati rice. Garnish with chopped fresh cilantro.

This turmeric chicken curry is full of bold, aromatic flavors from the blend of spices. The coconut milk adds a rich, creamy texture. Turmeric is known for its anti-inflammatory properties, making this a nutritious and delicious meal.

9. Brown Rice Pilaf with Almonds

Ingredients:
- 1 cup uncooked brown rice
- 2 cups low-sodium chicken or vegetable broth
- 1 tbsp olive oil
- 1 onion, diced
- 2 cloves garlic, minced
- 1 cup sliced mushrooms
- 1/2 cup slivered almonds
- 2 tbsp chopped fresh parsley
- 1 tsp dried thyme
- 1/2 tsp salt
- 1/4 tsp black pepper

Instructions:
1. In a medium saucepan, combine the uncooked brown rice and broth. Bring to a boil over high heat.

2. Once boiling, reduce heat to low, cover, and simmer for 25-30 minutes, until the rice is tender and the liquid is absorbed.

3. While the rice is cooking, heat the olive oil in a large skillet over medium heat. Add the diced onion and sauté for 3-4 minutes until translucent.

4. Add the minced garlic and sliced mushrooms to the skillet. Cook for 2-3 minutes more, until the mushrooms are softened.

5. Fluff the cooked brown rice with a fork and transfer it to the skillet with the onions and mushrooms.

6. Stir in the slivered almonds, chopped parsley, dried thyme, salt, and black pepper.

7. Cook the pilaf for 2-3 minutes, stirring frequently, to allow the flavors to meld.

8. Serve the brown rice pilaf warm, garnished with extra parsley if desired.

This brown rice pilaf is a delicious and nutritious side dish. The nutty brown rice, crunchy almonds, and earthy herbs and spices make it a flavorful accompaniment to grilled or roasted proteins. It's a simple yet satisfying way to enjoy whole grains.

10. Chickpea and Vegetable Stew

Ingredients:
- 2 tbsp olive oil
- 1 onion, diced
- 3 cloves garlic, minced
- 2 carrots, peeled and diced
- 2 celery stalks, diced
- 1 red bell pepper, diced
- 1 zucchini, diced
- 1 (15 oz) can chickpeas, drained and rinsed
- 1 (14.5 oz) can diced tomatoes
- 2 cups low-sodium vegetable broth
- 1 tsp dried thyme
- 1 tsp dried oregano
- 1/2 tsp smoked paprika
- Salt and black pepper to taste
- Chopped fresh parsley for garnish

Instructions:
1. In a large pot or Dutch oven, heat the olive oil over medium heat. Add the diced onion and sauté for 3-4 minutes until translucent.

2. Add the minced garlic and continue cooking for 1 minute, until fragrant.

3. Stir in the diced carrots, celery, bell pepper, and zucchini. Cook for 5-7 minutes, until the vegetables start to soften.

4. Add the drained and rinsed chickpeas, diced tomatoes, vegetable broth, dried thyme, dried oregano, and smoked paprika. Season with salt and black pepper to taste.

5. Bring the stew to a simmer, then reduce heat to medium-low. Let the stew simmer for 15-20 minutes, stirring occasionally, until the vegetables are tender.

6. Taste and adjust seasonings as needed.

7. Serve the chickpea and vegetable stew hot, garnished with chopped fresh parsley.

This hearty stew is packed with fiber-rich chickpeas and a variety of nutrient-dense vegetables. The blend of herbs and spices gives it great flavor. It's a comforting, one-pot meal that's perfect for a chilly day. Enjoy it on its own or serve it with crusty bread.

11. Ginger Garlic Shrimp Stir-Fry

Ingredients:
- 1 lb large shrimp, peeled and deveined
- 2 tbsp sesame oil, divided
- 3 cloves garlic, minced
- 1 tbsp grated fresh ginger
- 1 red bell pepper, sliced
- 1 cup snow peas or snap peas
- 2 green onions, sliced
- 2 tbsp low-sodium soy sauce
- 1 tbsp rice vinegar
- 1 tsp sesame seeds (optional)
- Salt and pepper to taste

Instructions:
1. Heat 1 tbsp of the sesame oil in a large skillet or wok over high heat.

2. Add the shrimp and cook for 2-3 minutes per side, until they just start to turn pink and curl up. Transfer the shrimp to a plate.

3. In the same skillet, heat the remaining 1 tbsp of sesame oil over medium-high heat. Add the minced garlic and grated ginger. Cook for 1 minute, stirring constantly, until fragrant.

4. Add the sliced red bell pepper and snow peas/snap peas to the skillet. Stir-fry for 3-4 minutes, until the vegetables are tender-crisp.

5. Return the cooked shrimp to the skillet. Add the soy sauce and rice vinegar. Toss everything together and cook for 2-3 minutes more, until the shrimp are fully cooked through.

6. Remove from heat and stir in the sliced green onions.

7. Serve the ginger garlic shrimp stir-fry immediately, garnished with sesame seeds if desired. Enjoy!

This shrimp stir-fry is bursting with bold Asian flavors from the ginger, garlic, and soy sauce. The crisp-tender vegetables and juicy shrimp make it a satisfying and nutritious meal. Serve it over steamed rice or noodles for a complete dish.

12. Baked Sweet Potato Fries

Ingredients:
- 2 lbs sweet potatoes, peeled and cut into 1/2-inch thick fry shapes
- 2 tbsp olive oil
- 1 tsp paprika
- 1 tsp garlic powder
- 1/2 tsp ground cumin
- 1/2 tsp salt
- 1/4 tsp black pepper

Instructions:

1. Preheat your oven to 400°F (200°C). Line a large baking sheet with parchment paper.

2. In a large bowl, toss the cut sweet potato fries with the olive oil, paprika, garlic powder, cumin, salt, and black pepper until the fries are evenly coated.

3. Spread the seasoned sweet potato fries in a single layer on the prepared baking sheet, making sure they are not touching each other.

4. Bake the fries in the preheated oven for 20 minutes. Flip the fries and continue baking for another 15-20 minutes, until they are crispy and lightly browned.

5. Remove the baked sweet potato fries from the oven and let them cool for a few minutes before serving.

Serving Suggestions:
- Serve the sweet potato fries as a side dish, or enjoy them as a healthy snack.
- For extra flavor, try dipping the fries in a creamy garlic aioli or a spicy sriracha mayo.
- Sprinkle the baked fries with grated parmesan cheese or chopped fresh herbs like rosemary or thyme.
- Add a dash of cayenne pepper or chili powder for a spicy twist.

These baked sweet potato fries are a delicious and nutritious alternative to traditional french fries. The combination of spices gives them a wonderful depth of flavor. Enjoy them as a guilt-free indulgence!

13. Avocado and Tomato Salad

Ingredients:
- 2 ripe avocados, diced
- 2 cups cherry or grape tomatoes, halved
- 1/2 red onion, thinly sliced
- 1/4 cup fresh basil leaves, chopped
- 2 tbsp olive oil
- 2 tbsp balsamic vinegar
- 1 tbsp fresh lemon juice
- 1/2 tsp salt
- 1/4 tsp black pepper

Instructions:

1. In a large bowl, gently combine the diced avocado, halved tomatoes, and sliced red onion.

2. Sprinkle the chopped fresh basil over the top.

3. In a small bowl, whisk together the olive oil, balsamic vinegar, lemon juice, salt, and black pepper.

4. Drizzle the vinaigrette over the avocado and tomato salad, and gently toss to coat.

5. Serve the salad immediately, or refrigerate for up to 30 minutes before serving to allow the flavors to meld.

Serving Suggestions:
- Serve the avocado and tomato salad as a side dish or light main course.

- Top the salad with grilled chicken or shrimp for a more substantial meal.

- Scoop the salad into halved avocado shells for a beautiful presentation.

- Sprinkle the salad with crumbled feta or shredded basil leaves for extra flavor.

This fresh and vibrant salad is a delicious way to enjoy the creamy texture of avocado paired with the juicy sweetness of tomatoes. The balsamic vinaigrette and fresh basil provide a perfect balance of flavors. It's a simple, healthy, and satisfying dish.

14. Steamed Asparagus with Lemon Butter

Ingredients:
- 1 lb fresh asparagus, trimmed
- 2 tbsp unsalted butter, softened
- 1 tbsp freshly squeezed lemon juice
- 1 tsp grated lemon zest
- 1/4 tsp salt
- 1/8 tsp black pepper

Instructions:

1. Fill a large pot with about 1 inch of water and bring it to a boil over high heat. Place a steamer basket in the pot.

2. Add the trimmed asparagus spears to the steamer basket. Cover the pot and steam the asparagus for 4-6 minutes, until tender-crisp.

3. While the asparagus is steaming, in a small bowl, combine the softened butter, lemon juice, lemon zest, salt, and black pepper. Mix well until fully incorporated.

4. Once the asparagus is cooked, transfer it to a serving plate. Immediately top the hot asparagus with the lemon butter mixture and gently toss to coat.

5. Serve the steamed asparagus with lemon butter immediately, while the butter is still melted.

Serving Suggestions:

- Sprinkle the asparagus with toasted sliced almonds or pine nuts for added crunch.

- Garnish with extra lemon zest or chopped fresh parsley.

- Serve the asparagus as a side dish to grilled or roasted meats, fish, or poultry.

- For a heartier meal, toss the asparagus with cooked pasta or quinoa.

This simple steamed asparagus dish is elevated by the bright, tangy lemon butter sauce. The lemon complements the natural sweetness of the asparagus perfectly. It's a quick and easy way to enjoy this nutritious spring vegetable.

15. Mediterranean Chickpea Salad

Ingredients:
- 1 (15 oz) can chickpeas, drained and rinsed
- 1 cup cherry tomatoes, halved
- 1/2 cup diced cucumber
- 1/4 cup diced red onion
- 1/4 cup crumbled feta cheese
- 2 tbsp chopped fresh parsley
- 2 tbsp chopped fresh basil
- 2 tbsp olive oil
- 1 tbsp red wine vinegar
- 1 tsp lemon juice
- 1/2 tsp dried oregano
- 1/4 tsp salt
- 1/8 tsp black pepper

Instructions:
1. In a large bowl, combine the drained and rinsed chickpeas, halved cherry tomatoes, diced cucumber, diced red onion, crumbled feta cheese, chopped parsley, and chopped basil.

2. In a small bowl, whisk together the olive oil, red wine vinegar, lemon juice, dried oregano, salt, and black pepper.

3. Pour the vinaigrette over the chickpea salad and toss gently to coat.

4. Cover the salad and refrigerate for at least 30 minutes to allow the flavors to meld.

5. Serve the chilled Mediterranean chickpea salad as a side dish or light main course.

Serving Suggestions:

- Scoop the salad onto a bed of mixed greens for a more substantial meal.

- Serve the chickpea salad with pita bread or crackers.

- Add grilled chicken or shrimp for extra protein.

- Garnish with additional fresh herbs or a sprinkle of za'atar seasoning.

This Mediterranean-inspired chickpea salad is packed with fresh, vibrant flavors from the tomatoes, cucumber, herbs, and tangy vinaigrette. The chickpeas provide fiber and plant-based protein, making it a nutritious and satisfying dish.

16. Roasted Cauliflower with Tahini Sauce

Ingredients:
For the Roasted Cauliflower:
- 1 head of cauliflower, cut into florets
- 2 tbsp olive oil
- 1 tsp ground cumin
- 1/2 tsp paprika
- 1/4 tsp salt
- 1/4 tsp black pepper

For the Tahini Sauce:
- 1/4 cup tahini (sesame seed paste)
- 2 tbsp freshly squeezed lemon juice
- 2 tbsp water
- 1 clove garlic, minced
- 1/4 tsp salt

Instructions:
1. Preheat your oven to 400°F (200°C). Line a large baking sheet with parchment paper.

2. In a large bowl, toss the cauliflower florets with the olive oil, cumin, paprika, salt, and black pepper until the cauliflower is evenly coated.

3. Spread the seasoned cauliflower in a single layer on the prepared baking sheet.

4. Roast the cauliflower in the preheated oven for 20-25 minutes, stirring halfway, until it is tender and lightly browned.

5. While the cauliflower is roasting, prepare the tahini sauce. In a small bowl, whisk together the tahini, lemon juice, water, minced garlic, and salt until smooth and creamy.

6. Once the roasted cauliflower is done, transfer it to a serving dish. Drizzle the tahini sauce over the top and gently toss to coat.

7. Serve the roasted cauliflower with tahini sauce warm or at room temperature.

Serving Suggestions:
- Sprinkle the roasted cauliflower with toasted sesame seeds or chopped fresh parsley for extra flavor and texture.
- Serve the cauliflower as a side dish or as part of a larger Mediterranean-inspired meal.
- The tahini sauce can also be used as a dip for raw vegetables or pita bread.

This roasted cauliflower dish is a delicious and nutritious way to enjoy this versatile vegetable. The creamy tahini sauce complements the nutty, earthy flavors of the roasted cauliflower perfectly.

17. Mushroom Barley Soup

Ingredients:
- 2 tbsp olive oil
- 1 onion, diced
- 3 cloves garlic, minced
- 8 oz cremini or
button mushrooms, sliced
- 1 cup pearl barley, rinsed
- 6 cups low-sodium vegetable
 or chicken broth
- 2 cups water
- 2 bay leaves
- 1 tsp dried thyme
- 1/2 tsp salt
- 1/4 tsp black pepper
- 2 cups chopped kale or spinach (optional)
- Chopped fresh parsley for garnish

Instructions:

1. In a large pot or Dutch oven, heat the olive oil over medium heat. Add the diced onion and sauté for 5 minutes until translucent.

2. Add the minced garlic and sliced mushrooms to the pot. Cook for 3-4 minutes, stirring occasionally, until the mushrooms are softened.

3. Stir in the rinsed pearl barley, vegetable or chicken broth, water, bay leaves, dried thyme, salt, and black pepper.

4. Bring the soup to a boil, then reduce heat to medium-low. Simmer for 25-30 minutes, stirring occasionally, until the barley is tender.

5. If using, stir in the chopped kale or spinach and cook for 2-3 minutes more, until the greens are wilted.

6. Remove the bay leaves. Taste the soup and adjust seasoning as needed. Serve the mushroom barley soup hot, garnished with chopped fresh parsley.

Variations:
- Add diced carrots, celery, or other vegetables to the soup.
- Use a mix of wild and cultivated mushrooms for extra flavor.
- Stir in a splash of sherry or dry white wine for depth.
- Top each bowl with shredded rotisserie chicken or crumbled feta cheese.

This hearty mushroom barley soup is packed with earthy, savory flavors. The pearl barley adds a wonderful chewy texture and makes it a satisfying, nutritious meal.

18. Grilled Vegetable Skewers

Ingredients:
- 1 red bell pepper, cut into 1-inch pieces
- 1 yellow squash, cut into 1-inch rounds
- 1 zucchini, cut into 1-inch rounds
- 1 red onion, cut into 1-inch pieces
- 8 oz cremini or button mushrooms, halved
- 2 tbsp olive oil
- 1 tsp dried oregano
- 1/2 tsp garlic powder
- 1/2 tsp salt
- 1/4 tsp black pepper

Instructions:
1. Preheat your grill to medium-high heat.

2. In a large bowl, combine the cut bell pepper, squash, zucchini, onion, and mushrooms. Drizzle with the olive oil and sprinkle with the dried oregano, garlic powder, salt, and black pepper. Toss to coat the vegetables evenly.

3. Thread the seasoned vegetables onto metal or wooden skewers, leaving a little space between each piece.

4. Grill the vegetable skewers for 12-15 minutes, turning occasionally, until the vegetables are tender and lightly charred.

5. Carefully remove the grilled vegetable skewers from the grill and serve immediately.

Serving Suggestions:
- Serve the grilled vegetable skewers as a side dish or a main course.
- Drizzle the skewers with a balsamic glaze or a lemon-herb vinaigrette.
- Sprinkle the grilled veggies with crumbled feta or shredded parmesan cheese.
- Serve the skewers over a bed of quinoa or couscous for a more substantial meal.
- Offer any leftover grilled vegetables as a topping for salads or sandwiches.

These colorful and flavorful grilled vegetable skewers are a great way to enjoy a variety of fresh produce. The high-heat grilling brings out the natural sweetness of the vegetables and adds a delicious smoky char.

19. Lemon Herb Baked Cod

Ingredients:
- 1 lb cod fillets
- 2 tbsp olive oil
- 2 tbsp freshly squeezed lemon juice
- 2 tsp grated lemon zest
- 2 tbsp chopped fresh parsley
- 1 tbsp chopped fresh dill
- 1 tsp dried thyme
- 1/2 tsp salt
- 1/4 tsp black pepper

Instructions:

1. Preheat your oven to 400°F (200°C). Lightly grease a baking dish or line it with parchment paper.

2. Place the cod fillets in the prepared baking dish.

3. In a small bowl, whisk together the olive oil, lemon juice, lemon zest, parsley, dill, thyme, salt, and black pepper.

4. Drizzle the lemon herb mixture over the cod fillets, making sure to evenly coat the fish.

5. Bake the cod in the preheated oven for 15-20 minutes, or until the fish flakes easily with a fork and is opaque throughout.

6. Remove the baked cod from the oven and serve immediately, garnished with additional fresh herbs if desired.

Serving Suggestions:
- Serve the lemon herb baked cod with roasted vegetables, steamed rice, or a fresh salad.
- For a heartier meal, top the cod with sautéed spinach or a dollop of pesto.
- Squeeze extra lemon juice over the top of the fish just before serving.
- Sprinkle the baked cod with toasted breadcrumbs or sliced almonds for added texture.

This simple baked cod recipe is packed with bright, fresh flavors from the lemon, herbs, and olive oil. The cod fillets come out tender and flaky every time. It's a quick and easy way to enjoy a healthy, delicious seafood dish.

20. Cucumber and Feta Salad

Ingredients:
- 2 English cucumbers, sliced into half-moons
- 1 cup cherry or grape tomatoes, halved
- 1/2 red onion, thinly sliced
- 1/2 cup crumbled feta cheese
- 2 tbsp chopped fresh dill
- 2 tbsp olive oil
- 1 tbsp red wine vinegar
- 1 tbsp freshly squeezed lemon juice
- 1/2 tsp dried oregano
- 1/4 tsp salt
- 1/8 tsp black pepper

Instructions:

1. In a large bowl, combine the sliced cucumbers, halved tomatoes, and thinly sliced red onion.

2. Sprinkle the crumbled feta cheese and chopped fresh dill over the top of the vegetables.

3. In a small bowl, whisk together the olive oil, red wine vinegar, lemon juice, dried oregano, salt, and black pepper.

4. Drizzle the vinaigrette over the cucumber and feta salad, and gently toss to coat.

5. Cover the salad and refrigerate for at least 30 minutes to allow the flavors to meld.

6. Serve the chilled cucumber and feta salad as a side dish or light main course.

Serving Suggestions:
- Add grilled chicken or shrimp to turn this salad into a more substantial meal.
- Serve the salad on a bed of mixed greens or over quinoa or couscous.
- Garnish with additional fresh dill, lemon wedges, or a sprinkle of za'atar seasoning.
- For a creamier texture, stir in a tablespoon or two of Greek yogurt.

This refreshing cucumber and feta salad is a perfect side dish for warm weather. The crisp cucumbers, juicy tomatoes, and tangy feta are complemented by the bright, herbal vinaigrette. It's a light, flavorful, and nutritious option.

21. Spaghetti Squash with Marinara Sauce

Ingredients:
- 1 medium spaghetti squash, halved lengthwise and seeds removed
- 1 tbsp olive oil
- 1/2 tsp salt
- 1/4 tsp black pepper
- 1 (24 oz) jar marinara sauce
- 1/4 cup grated parmesan cheese (optional)
- Chopped fresh basil for garnish

Instructions:

1. Preheat your oven to 400°F (200°C). Line a baking sheet with parchment paper.

2. Place the spaghetti squash halves cut-side up on the prepared baking sheet. Drizzle the squash with the olive oil and season with salt and pepper.

3. Roast the spaghetti squash in the preheated oven for 40-50 minutes, until the flesh is tender and easily separates into spaghetti-like strands when scraped with a fork.

4. Remove the roasted spaghetti squash from the oven and let it cool for 5-10 minutes.

5. Using a fork, gently scrape the flesh of the spaghetti squash into a bowl, separating the strands.

6. In a saucepan, heat the marinara sauce over medium heat until warmed through.

7. Serve the spaghetti squash strands topped with the warm marinara sauce. Sprinkle with grated parmesan cheese and chopped fresh basil, if desired.

Serving Suggestions:
- For a heartier meal, top the spaghetti squash with grilled chicken, meatballs, or sautéed vegetables.
- Mix in some pesto or a drizzle of olive oil and garlic for extra flavor.
- Swap the marinara sauce for a creamy alfredo or pesto sauce.
- Serve the spaghetti squash with a side salad or garlic bread for a complete meal.

This spaghetti squash dish is a delicious and nutritious alternative to traditional pasta. The roasted squash strands have a similar texture to spaghetti, making it a great low-carb option.

22. Baked Apples with Cinnamon

Ingredients:
- 4 medium-sized apples (such as Gala, Honeycrisp, or Fuji)
- 1/4 cup brown sugar
- 2 tsp ground cinnamon
- 2 tbsp unsalted butter, softened
- 1/4 cup chopped walnuts or pecans (optional)
- Vanilla ice cream or whipped cream for serving (optional)

Instructions:

1. Preheat your oven to 375°F (190°C). Lightly grease a baking dish or line it with parchment paper.

2. Wash and core the apples, leaving a small well in the center of each one. Place the apples in the prepared baking dish.

3. In a small bowl, mix together the brown sugar and ground cinnamon.

4. Stuff the center of each apple with about 1 tbsp of the cinnamon-sugar mixture. Top each apple with a small pat of the softened butter.

5. If using, sprinkle the chopped walnuts or pecans around the base of the apples in the baking dish.

6. Bake the stuffed apples in the preheated oven for 30-40 minutes, or until the apples are tender when pierced with a fork and the filling is bubbly.

7. Remove the baked apples from the oven and let them cool for 5-10 minutes.

8. Serve the warm baked apples with a scoop of vanilla ice cream or a dollop of whipped cream, if desired.

Variations:
- For a different flavor, try using oats, raisins, or dried cranberries in the filling.
- Drizzle the baked apples with a caramel or maple sauce.
- Sprinkle the apples with a pinch of nutmeg or allspice along with the cinnamon.

These baked apples make a delightful and comforting dessert. The sweet, cinnamon-spiced filling complements the soft, tender apples perfectly. It's a simple yet satisfying way to enjoy the flavors of fall.

23. Miso Glazed Eggplant

Ingredients:
- 2 medium eggplants, cut into 1-inch thick slices
- 2 tbsp white or yellow miso paste
- 2 tbsp mirin
- 1 tbsp rice vinegar
- 1 tbsp honey
- 1 tsp sesame oil
- 1 tsp grated fresh ginger
- 1 tsp sesame seeds (optional)
- Chopped green onions for garnish (optional)

Instructions:

1. Preheat your oven to 400°F (200°C). Line a baking sheet with parchment paper.

2. Arrange the eggplant slices in a single layer on the prepared baking sheet.

3. In a small bowl, whisk together the miso paste, mirin, rice vinegar, honey, sesame oil, and grated ginger until well combined.

4. Brush the miso glaze generously over the top of the eggplant slices, making sure to coat them evenly.

5. Bake the miso glazed eggplant in the preheated oven for 20-25 minutes, flipping the slices halfway through, until the eggplant is tender and the glaze is caramelized.

6. Remove the baked eggplant from the oven and sprinkle with sesame seeds, if using.

7. Serve the miso glazed eggplant warm, garnished with chopped green onions.

Serving Suggestions:
- Serve the eggplant as a side dish or as part of a larger Asian-inspired meal.
- Toss the baked eggplant with cooked rice or quinoa for a more substantial dish.
- Drizzle the eggplant with a bit of soy sauce or sriracha for extra flavor.
- Pair the miso glazed eggplant with grilled or roasted proteins like salmon, chicken, or tofu.

The sweet and savory miso glaze creates a delicious caramelized coating on the tender eggplant. This simple yet flavorful dish is a great way to enjoy this versatile vegetable.

24. Broccoli and Quinoa Salad

Ingredients:
- 1 cup uncooked quinoa, rinsed
- 2 cups low-sodium vegetable or chicken broth
- 2 cups broccoli florets, chopped into bite-size pieces
- 1/2 cup diced red bell pepper
- 1/4 cup diced red onion
- 2 tbsp chopped fresh parsley
- 2 tbsp chopped fresh basil
- 2 tbsp olive oil
- 1 tbsp lemon juice
- 1 tsp Dijon mustard
- 1/2 tsp salt
- 1/4 tsp black pepper

Instructions:
1. In a medium saucepan, combine the rinsed quinoa and broth. Bring to a boil over high heat.

2. Once boiling, reduce the heat to low, cover, and simmer for 15-20 minutes, until the quinoa is tender and the liquid is absorbed. Fluff the quinoa with a fork and let it cool slightly.

3. In a large bowl, combine the cooked quinoa, chopped broccoli florets, diced red bell pepper, diced red onion, chopped parsley, and chopped basil.

4. In a small bowl, whisk together the olive oil, lemon juice, Dijon mustard, salt, and black pepper to make the dressing.

5. Pour the dressing over the quinoa and vegetable mixture and toss gently to coat. Serve the broccoli and quinoa salad chilled or at room temperature.

Serving Suggestions:
- Add grilled chicken or shrimp to turn this salad into a main dish.
- Sprinkle the salad with toasted slivered almonds or sunflower seeds for extra crunch.
- Swap the basil for other fresh herbs like cilantro or dill.
- Stir in a handful of crumbled feta or shredded cheddar cheese.

This broccoli and quinoa salad is a nutritious and flavorful side dish or light main course. The combination of protein-rich quinoa, crunchy broccoli, and fresh herbs makes it a satisfying and wholesome option.

25. Grilled Turkey Burgers

Ingredients:
- 1 lb ground turkey
- 1/4 cup finely chopped onion
- 2 cloves garlic, minced
- 1 tsp dried oregano
- 1/2 tsp salt
- 1/4 tsp black pepper
- 4 whole wheat burger buns
- Toppings of your choice (e.g., lettuce, tomato, avocado, cheese, etc.)

Instructions:
1. Preheat your grill to medium-high heat.

2. In a large bowl, gently mix together the ground turkey, chopped onion, minced garlic, dried oregano, salt, and black pepper until just combined. Be careful not to overmix.

3. Divide the turkey mixture into 4 equal portions and shape them into patties, each about 4-5 inches wide and 1/2 inch thick.

4. Lightly oil the grill grates to prevent the burgers from sticking.

5. Grill the turkey burgers for 4-5 minutes per side, or until they are cooked through and reach an internal temperature of 165°F (75°C).

6. Toast the burger buns on the grill for 1-2 minutes, if desired.

7. Place the grilled turkey burgers on the toasted buns and top with your desired toppings.

Serving Suggestions:
- Serve the turkey burgers with a side of grilled vegetables, a fresh salad, or baked sweet potato fries.
- Top the burgers with sliced avocado, sautéed mushrooms, or caramelized onions for extra flavor.
- For a spicy twist, add a dollop of chipotle mayo or a sprinkle of cayenne pepper.
- Swap the whole wheat buns for lettuce wraps or portobello mushroom caps for a low-carb option.

These juicy, flavorful grilled turkey burgers are a healthier alternative to traditional beef burgers. The combination of lean turkey, aromatic herbs, and your favorite toppings makes for a delicious and satisfying meal.

26. Kale and White Bean Soup

Ingredients:
- 2 tbsp olive oil
- 1 onion, diced
- 3 cloves garlic, minced
- 2 carrots, peeled and diced
- 2 celery stalks, diced
- 1 tsp dried thyme
- 1/2 tsp dried rosemary
- 1/4 tsp red pepper flakes (optional)
- 4 cups low-sodium vegetable or chicken broth
- 1 (15 oz) can white beans, drained and rinsed
- 4 cups chopped kale, stems removed
- 1 tsp salt
- 1/4 tsp black pepper

Instructions:

1. In a large pot or Dutch oven, heat the olive oil over medium heat. Add the diced onion and sauté for 3-4 minutes until translucent.

2. Add the minced garlic, diced carrots, and diced celery. Cook for 2-3 minutes, stirring frequently, until fragrant.

3. Stir in the dried thyme, dried rosemary, and red pepper flakes (if using). Cook for 1 minute.

4. Pour in the vegetable or chicken broth and add the drained and rinsed white beans. Bring the soup to a simmer.

5. Add the chopped kale to the pot and cook for 5-7 minutes, until the kale is tender. Season the soup with salt and black pepper to taste.

6. Serve the kale and white bean soup hot, garnished with additional black pepper or a drizzle of olive oil, if desired.

Variations:
- Use cannellini, navy, or Great Northern beans instead of white beans.
- Add diced potatoes or cooked pasta for extra heartiness.
- Stir in a splash of lemon juice or sherry vinegar for brightness.
- Top the soup with grated parmesan cheese or crumbled feta.

This nourishing kale and white bean soup is packed with fiber, protein, and vitamins. The combination of tender kale, creamy beans, and aromatic vegetables makes it a comforting and satisfying meal.

27. Stuffed Bell Peppers with Turkey and Quinoa

Ingredients:
- 1 tsp dried oregano
- 1/2 tsp ground cumin
- 1/2 tsp salt
- 1/4 tsp black pepper
- 1 cup marinara sauce
- 1/2 cup shredded mozzarella cheese
- 4 bell peppers (any color), halved lengthwise and seeds removed
- 1 cup cooked quinoa
- 1 lb ground turkey
- 1 onion, diced
- 2 cloves garlic, minced

Instructions:

1. Preheat your oven to 375°F (190°C). Lightly grease a baking dish or line it with parchment paper.

2. Arrange the bell pepper halves, cut-side up, in the prepared baking dish.

3. In a large skillet over medium heat, cook the ground turkey, diced onion, and minced garlic until the turkey is browned and the onion is translucent, about 5-7 minutes. Drain any excess fat.

4. Stir in the cooked quinoa, dried oregano, ground cumin, salt, and black pepper. Mix well to combine.

5. Spoon the turkey and quinoa mixture evenly into the bell pepper halves, pressing it down gently.

6. Pour the marinara sauce over the stuffed peppers, making sure to coat the tops.

7. Cover the baking dish with foil and bake in the preheated oven for 30 minutes.

8. Remove the foil, sprinkle the shredded mozzarella cheese over the tops of the stuffed peppers, and bake for an additional 10-15 minutes, until the cheese is melted and bubbly. Serve the stuffed bell peppers hot, garnished with fresh basil or parsley if desired.

Variations:
- Use a mixture of ground turkey and ground beef for a heartier filling.
- Swap the quinoa for cooked brown rice or farro.
- Add sautéed mushrooms, spinach, or diced tomatoes to the filling.
- Top the stuffed peppers with grated parmesan or crumbled feta cheese.

These stuffed bell peppers are a delicious and nutritious meal. The combination of lean turkey, quinoa, and vegetables makes for a satisfying and flavorful dish.

28. Lemon Garlic Shrimp Pasta

Ingredients:
- 8 oz whole wheat or gluten-free pasta (such as spaghetti or linguine)
- 1 lb large shrimp, peeled and deveined
- 2 tbsp olive oil
- 3 cloves garlic, minced
- 1/4 cup dry white wine or low-sodium chicken broth
- 2 tbsp freshly squeezed lemon juice
- 1 tsp grated lemon zest
- 1/4 cup chopped fresh parsley
- 1/4 tsp red pepper flakes (optional)
- Salt and black pepper to taste

Instructions:
1. Bring a large pot of salted water to a boil. Cook the whole wheat or gluten-free pasta according to the package instructions until al dente. Drain and set aside.

2. In a large skillet, heat the olive oil over medium-high heat. Add the shrimp and minced garlic. Cook for 2-3 minutes, stirring frequently, until the shrimp start to turn pink.

3. Deglaze the pan by pouring in the white wine or chicken broth. Scrape up any browned bits from the bottom of the pan.

4. Stir in the freshly squeezed lemon juice, lemon zest, chopped parsley, and red pepper flakes (if using). Season with salt and black pepper to taste.

5. Add the cooked pasta to the skillet and toss everything together until the pasta is well coated and heated through, about 2-3 minutes.

6. Serve the lemon garlic shrimp pasta immediately, garnished with additional parsley if desired.

Variations:
- Use whole grain or gluten-free penne, fusilli, or farfalle instead of spaghetti or linguine.
- Add sautéed spinach, cherry tomatoes, or zucchini noodles to the pasta.
- Sprinkle the dish with grated parmesan or crumbled feta cheese.
- For a creamier sauce, stir in a tablespoon or two of heavy cream or Greek yogurt.

This lemon garlic shrimp pasta is a light, flavorful, and nutritious meal. The whole wheat or gluten-free pasta provides complex carbohydrates, while the shrimp adds lean protein. It's a delicious and easy-to-prepare dish that's perfect for a weeknight dinner.

29. Ratatouille

Ingredients:
- 1 medium eggplant, cut into 1-inch cubes
- 1 medium zucchini, halved lengthwise and sliced 1/2-inch thick
- 1 medium yellow squash, halved lengthwise and sliced 1/2-inch thick
- 1 red bell pepper, seeded and cut into 1-inch pieces
- 1 yellow onion, halved and thinly sliced
- 3 garlic cloves, minced
- 2 tablespoons olive oil
- 1 (14.5 oz) can diced tomatoes
- 1 teaspoon dried thyme
- 1 teaspoon dried oregano
- Salt and freshly ground black pepper to taste
- 2 tablespoons chopped fresh basil

Instructions:

1. In a large skillet or Dutch oven, heat the olive oil over medium-high heat. Add the eggplant, zucchini, squash, bell pepper, onion, and garlic. Cook, stirring occasionally, until the vegetables are tender, about 10-12 minutes.

2. Add the diced tomatoes, thyme, oregano, salt, and pepper. Stir to combine.

3. Reduce heat to medium-low and simmer for 15-20 minutes, stirring occasionally, until the vegetables are very soft and the flavors have melded.

4. Remove from heat and stir in the fresh basil.

5. Serve warm or at room temperature. Ratatouille can be served as a side dish or as a main course over pasta, rice, or crusty bread.

30. Cauliflower Rice Stir–Fry

Ingredients:
- 1 head of cauliflower, cut into florets
- 2 tablespoons olive oil
- 1 onion, diced
- 3 cloves garlic, minced
- 1 inch piece of ginger, grated
- 1 red bell pepper, diced
- 1 cup sliced mushrooms
- 2 cups baby spinach
- 2 tablespoons soy sauce
- 1 tablespoon rice vinegar
- 1 teaspoon sesame oil
- Salt and pepper to taste
- Chopped green onions and sesame seeds for garnish (optional)

Instructions:
1. In a food processor, pulse the cauliflower florets until they resemble rice or couscous. Set aside.

2. Heat the olive oil in a large skillet or wok over medium-high heat. Add the onion and sauté for 2-3 minutes until translucent.

3. Add the garlic and ginger and cook for 1 minute, until fragrant.

4. Add the bell pepper and mushrooms. Stir-fry for 3-4 minutes until the vegetables are tender-crisp.

5. Add the cauliflower rice to the pan. Stir-fry for 5-7 minutes, until the cauliflower is tender but still has a bit of bite.

6. Stir in the spinach, soy sauce, rice vinegar, and sesame oil. Cook for 1-2 minutes until the spinach is wilted.

7. Season with salt and pepper to taste.

8. Serve the cauliflower rice stir-fry hot, garnished with chopped green onions and sesame seeds if desired.

This makes a great low-carb, veggie-packed meal! Let me know if you have any other questions.

31. Walnut Crusted Baked Chicken

Ingredients:
- 4 boneless, skinless chicken breasts
- 1 cup chopped walnuts
- 1/2 cup panko breadcrumbs
- 2 tablespoons grated Parmesan cheese
- 1 teaspoon dried thyme
- 1/2 teaspoon garlic powder
- 1/4 teaspoon salt
- 1/4 teaspoon black pepper
- 2 tablespoons olive oil

Instructions:

1. Preheat your oven to 400°F (200°C). Line a baking sheet with parchment paper or a silicone baking mat.

2. In a food processor, pulse the walnuts until they are finely chopped, but not turned into a powder. Transfer the chopped walnuts to a shallow bowl.

3. In the same bowl, mix together the panko breadcrumbs, Parmesan cheese, thyme, garlic powder, salt, and black pepper.

4. Brush the chicken breasts lightly with the olive oil on both sides.

5. Dip the chicken breasts into the walnut mixture, pressing gently to help the coating adhere. Place the coated chicken breasts on the prepared baking sheet.

6. Bake the chicken for 25-30 minutes, or until the internal temperature reaches 165°F (75°C) and the coating is golden brown.

7. Remove the chicken from the oven and let it rest for 5 minutes before serving.

Serve the walnut crusted baked chicken warm, garnished with fresh herbs or a lemon wedge if desired. This dish pairs well with roasted vegetables, a fresh salad, or your favorite side dish.

32. Greek Salad with Feta Cheese

Ingredients:
- 1 head romaine lettuce, chopped
- 1 cucumber, diced
- 1 pint cherry tomatoes, halved
- 1 red onion, thinly sliced
- 1 cup kalamata olives, pitted and halved
- 1 cup crumbled feta cheese
- 2 tablespoons olive oil
- 2 tablespoons red wine vinegar
- 1 teaspoon dried oregano
- 1/2 teaspoon salt
- 1/4 teaspoon black pepper

Instructions:
1. In a large salad bowl, combine the chopped romaine lettuce, diced cucumber, halved cherry tomatoes, thinly sliced red onion, and halved kalamata olives.

2. Sprinkle the crumbled feta cheese over the top of the salad.

3. In a small bowl, whisk together the olive oil, red wine vinegar, dried oregano, salt, and black pepper to make the dressing.

4. Drizzle the dressing over the salad and gently toss to coat everything evenly.

5. Serve the Greek salad immediately, or refrigerate until ready to serve. The flavors will meld together as it chills.

Optional add-ins:
- Grilled or roasted chicken for a heartier meal
- Pepperoncini peppers
- Garbanzo beans or chickpeas
- Sliced bell peppers

This fresh and flavorful Greek salad makes a wonderful light lunch or side dish. The combination of crisp vegetables, briny olives, tangy feta, and the simple vinaigrette dressing is simply delicious. Enjoy!

33. Tofu and Vegetable Curry

Ingredients:
- 1 block (14 oz) extra-firm tofu, cubed
- 2 tablespoons coconut oil
- 1 onion, diced
- 3 cloves garlic, minced
- 1 tablespoon grated fresh ginger
- 2 tablespoons curry powder
- 1 teaspoon ground cumin
- 1 teaspoon ground coriander
- 1/4 teaspoon cayenne pepper (or to taste)
- 1 red bell pepper, sliced
- 1 cup cauliflower florets
- 1 cup baby spinach
- 1 (13.5 oz) can coconut milk
- 1 tablespoon soy sauce or tamari
- Salt and pepper to taste
- Chopped cilantro for garnish

Instructions:

1. Press the tofu block between paper towels or a clean kitchen towel to remove excess moisture. Cut into 1-inch cubes.

2. In a large skillet or wok, heat the coconut oil over medium heat. Add the cubed tofu and cook, stirring occasionally, until lightly browned on all sides, about 5-7 minutes. Transfer the tofu to a plate.

3. In the same skillet, add the diced onion and sauté for 3-4 minutes until translucent. Add the garlic and ginger and cook for 1 minute more, until fragrant.

4. Stir in the curry powder, cumin, coriander, and cayenne. Cook for 1 minute to toast the spices.

5. Add the sliced bell pepper and cauliflower florets. Sauté for 5 minutes, until the vegetables start to soften.

6. Pour in the coconut milk and soy sauce. Bring the mixture to a simmer and cook for 5-7 minutes, until the vegetables are tender.

7. Gently stir the cooked tofu and baby spinach into the curry. Cook for 2-3 minutes until the spinach is wilted.

8. Season with salt and pepper to taste. Serve the tofu and vegetable curry over steamed rice, garnished with chopped cilantro.

34. Butternut Squash Soup

Ingredients:
- 1 medium butternut squash, peeled, seeded, and cubed (about 4 cups)
- 1 onion, diced
- 2 cloves garlic, minced
- 2 tablespoons olive oil
- 4 cups vegetable or chicken broth
- 1 cup milk or unsweetened almond milk
- 1 teaspoon ground cumin
- 1/2 teaspoon ground cinnamon
- 1/4 teaspoon ground nutmeg
- Salt and pepper to taste
- Chopped fresh parsley or thyme for garnish (optional)

Instructions:

1. In a large pot or Dutch oven, heat the olive oil over medium heat. Add the diced onion and sauté for 5 minutes until translucent.

2. Add the minced garlic and sauté for 1 minute more, until fragrant.

3. Add the cubed butternut squash and vegetable/chicken broth. Bring the mixture to a boil.

4. Reduce the heat to medium-low, cover the pot, and simmer for 20-25 minutes, until the squash is very soft.

5. Remove the pot from the heat and use an immersion blender to puree the soup until smooth and creamy. Alternatively, you can carefully transfer the soup to a blender in batches and blend until smooth.

6. Stir in the milk or almond milk, cumin, cinnamon, and nutmeg. Season with salt and pepper to taste.

7. Return the soup to low heat and cook for 5 more minutes, stirring occasionally, to allow the flavors to meld.

8. Ladle the butternut squash soup into bowls and garnish with chopped fresh parsley or thyme, if desired.

Serve the soup warm, with crusty bread or a salad on the side. The sweet and savory flavors of the butternut squash make this soup so comforting and delicious

35. Zucchini Noodles with Pesto

Ingredients:
- 3 medium zucchinis, spiralized or julienned into noodles
- 1 cup fresh basil leaves
- 1/4 cup pine nuts
- 2 cloves garlic
- 1/4 cup grated Parmesan cheese
- 2 tablespoons olive oil
- 1 tablespoon lemon juice
- Salt and pepper to taste

Instructions:

1. Make the pesto: In a food processor or blender, combine the fresh basil leaves, pine nuts, garlic, Parmesan cheese, olive oil, and lemon juice. Pulse until a smooth pesto forms. Season with salt and pepper to taste.

2. Prepare the zucchini noodles: Use a spiralizer, julienne peeler, or mandoline slicer to cut the zucchinis into long, thin noodle-like strips.

3. In a large skillet or wok, heat the zucchini noodles over medium heat for 2-3 minutes, just until they start to soften slightly. Be careful not to overcook them or they will become watery.

4. Remove the zucchini noodles from the heat and transfer them to a serving bowl.

5. Add the prepared pesto to the zucchini noodles and toss gently to coat the noodles evenly.

6. Serve the zucchini noodles with pesto immediately, garnished with extra Parmesan cheese, pine nuts, or fresh basil leaves if desired.

The fresh, vibrant pesto pairs perfectly with the tender zucchini noodles for a light and healthy meal. You can also add grilled chicken, shrimp, or roasted vegetables to make it more substantial.

36. Baked Cod with Tomato and Olive Relish

Ingredients:
For the Tomato and Olive Relish:
- 1 cup cherry tomatoes, halved
- 1/2 cup pitted kalamata olives, chopped
- 2 tablespoons chopped fresh parsley
- 1 tablespoon olive oil
- 1 tablespoon red wine vinegar
- 1 garlic clove, minced
- Salt and pepper to taste

For the Baked Cod:
- 4 (6 oz) cod fillets
- 2 tablespoons olive oil
- 1 teaspoon paprika
- 1/2 teaspoon dried oregano
- Salt and pepper to taste

Instructions:
1. Make the tomato and olive relish: In a medium bowl, combine the halved cherry tomatoes, chopped kalamata olives, chopped parsley, olive oil, red wine vinegar, and minced garlic. Season with salt and pepper to taste. Set aside.

2. Preheat your oven to 400°F (200°C). Line a baking sheet with parchment paper or foil.

3. Pat the cod fillets dry with paper towels and place them on the prepared baking sheet. Drizzle the cod with the 2 tablespoons of olive oil and sprinkle with paprika, dried oregano, salt, and pepper.

4. Bake the cod for 12-15 minutes, or until it flakes easily with a fork and reaches an internal temperature of 145°F (63°C).

5. Remove the baked cod from the oven and transfer the fillets to serving plates.

6. Top each piece of cod with a generous spoonful of the tomato and olive relish.

7. Serve the baked cod with the tomato and olive relish immediately, garnished with extra chopped parsley if desired.

The bright, tangy relish complements the mild, flaky cod perfectly. This dish is a healthy and delicious way to enjoy seafood. Enjoy!

37. Arugula and Orange Salad with Goat Cheese

Ingredients:
- 5 oz baby arugula
- 2 navel oranges, peeled and segmented
- 1/2 cup crumbled goat cheese
- 1/4 cup toasted sliced almonds
- 2 tablespoons olive oil
- 1 tablespoon white wine vinegar
- 1 teaspoon Dijon mustard
- 1 teaspoon honey
- Salt and pepper to taste

Instructions:

1. In a large salad bowl, combine the baby arugula, orange segments, crumbled goat cheese, and toasted sliced almonds.

2. In a small bowl, whisk together the olive oil, white wine vinegar, Dijon mustard, and honey until emulsified. Season the dressing with salt and pepper to taste.

3. Drizzle the dressing over the salad and gently toss to coat the greens and other ingredients evenly.

4. Serve the arugula and orange salad immediately.

Tips:
- To segment the oranges, use a sharp knife to cut off the top and bottom of the fruit. Then, cut away the peel and white pith, following the curve of the fruit. Slice between the membranes to release the orange segments.

- Toast the sliced almonds in a dry skillet over medium heat for 2-3 minutes, stirring frequently, until fragrant and lightly browned.

- For a heartier meal, you can add grilled chicken or shrimp to the salad.

The peppery arugula, sweet oranges, tangy goat cheese, and crunchy almonds make this salad a delightful balance of flavors and textures. Enjoy this fresh and vibrant salad!

38. Black Bean and Corn Salad

Ingredients:
- 1 (15 oz) can black beans, rinsed and drained
- 1 (15 oz) can corn, drained
- 1 red bell pepper, diced
- 1 cup cherry tomatoes, halved
- 1/2 red onion, diced
- 1/4 cup chopped fresh cilantro
- 2 tablespoons olive oil
- 2 tablespoons lime juice
- 1 teaspoon ground cumin
- 1/2 teaspoon chili powder
- Salt and pepper to taste

Instructions:
1. In a large bowl, combine the rinsed and drained black beans, drained corn, diced red bell pepper, halved cherry tomatoes, and diced red onion.

2. Add the chopped fresh cilantro to the bowl.

3. In a small bowl, whisk together the olive oil, lime juice, ground cumin, and chili powder. Season the dressing with salt and pepper to taste.

4. Pour the dressing over the black bean and corn salad and toss gently to coat everything evenly.

5. Cover the salad and refrigerate for at least 30 minutes to allow the flavors to meld.

6. Serve the black bean and corn salad chilled or at room temperature.

This salad makes a great side dish or a light main course. It's packed with protein from the black beans, fiber, and a variety of fresh vegetables. The tangy lime dressing complements the sweetness of the corn and the subtle heat from the chili powder.

You can customize this salad by adding other ingredients like avocado, jalapeño, or crumbled feta cheese. It's also delicious served with tortilla chips or over a bed of greens.

39. Ginger Soy Glazed Salmon

Ingredients:
- 4 (6 oz) salmon fillets
- 2 tablespoons soy sauce
- 2 tablespoons honey
- 1 tablespoon rice vinegar
- 1 tablespoon grated fresh ginger
- 1 clove garlic, minced
- 1/4 teaspoon red pepper flakes (optional)
- Salt and pepper to taste
- Chopped green onions for garnish (optional)

Instructions:

1. Preheat your oven to 400°F (200°C). Line a baking sheet with parchment paper or foil.

2. In a small bowl, whisk together the soy sauce, honey, rice vinegar, grated ginger, minced garlic, and red pepper flakes (if using). Season with a pinch of salt and pepper.

3. Place the salmon fillets skin-side down on the prepared baking sheet. Brush the tops and sides of the salmon with the ginger soy glaze, reserving any extra glaze.

4. Bake the salmon for 12-15 minutes, or until it flakes easily with a fork and reaches an internal temperature of 145°F (63°C).

5. Remove the salmon from the oven and brush the fillets with any remaining ginger soy glaze.

6. Serve the ginger soy glazed salmon immediately, garnished with chopped green onions if desired.

This salmon dish is full of bold, Asian-inspired flavors. The sweet and savory glaze caramelizes on the salmon as it bakes, creating a delicious crust.

Serve the salmon with steamed rice, roasted vegetables, or a fresh salad for a complete and healthy meal. Enjoy!

40. Chickpea and Spinach Curry

Ingredients:
- 2 tablespoons olive oil
- 1 onion, diced
- 3 cloves garlic, minced
- 1 tablespoon grated fresh ginger
- 2 teaspoons garam masala
- 1 teaspoon ground cumin
- 1 teaspoon ground coriander
- 1/4 teaspoon cayenne pepper (or to taste)
- 1 (15 oz) can chickpeas, rinsed and drained
- 1 (14 oz) can diced tomatoes
- 1 cup vegetable broth
- 5 oz baby spinach
- 1/4 cup full-fat coconut milk
- Salt and pepper to taste
- Chopped cilantro for garnish

Instructions:
1. In a large skillet or Dutch oven, heat the olive oil over medium heat. Add the diced onion and sauté for 5 minutes until translucent.

2. Add the minced garlic and grated ginger. Cook for 1 minute, until fragrant.

3. Stir in the garam masala, cumin, coriander, and cayenne pepper. Cook for 1 minute to toast the spices.

4. Add the rinsed and drained chickpeas, diced tomatoes, and vegetable broth. Bring the mixture to a simmer.

5. Reduce the heat to medium-low and let the curry simmer for 10-15 minutes, stirring occasionally, until slightly thickened.

6. Stir in the baby spinach and coconut milk. Cook for 2-3 minutes, until the spinach is wilted.

7. Season the chickpea and spinach curry with salt and pepper to taste. Serve the curry hot, garnished with chopped fresh cilantro. Enjoy with basmati rice or naan bread.

This vegetarian curry is packed with protein from the chickpeas and nutrients from the spinach. The blend of aromatic spices creates a delicious, complex flavor. Adjust the cayenne pepper to your desired level of heat.

41. Quinoa Stuffed Portobello Mushrooms

Ingredients:
- 4 large portobello mushroom caps, stems removed and chopped
- 1 cup cooked quinoa
- 1/2 cup diced tomatoes
- 1/2 cup crumbled feta cheese
- 1/4 cup chopped fresh basil
- 2 cloves garlic, minced
- 1 tablespoon olive oil
- Salt and pepper to taste

Instructions:

1. Preheat your oven to 400°F (200°C). Line a baking sheet with parchment paper.

2. Gently wipe the portobello mushroom caps clean with a damp paper towel. Remove the stems and chop them finely.

3. In a medium bowl, combine the chopped mushroom stems, cooked quinoa, diced tomatoes, crumbled feta cheese, chopped basil, and minced garlic. Stir to mix well.

4. Brush the portobello mushroom caps lightly with the olive oil and place them on the prepared baking sheet, gill-side up.

5. Divide the quinoa stuffing mixture evenly among the mushroom caps, piling it up in the center.

6. Bake the stuffed portobello mushrooms for 15-20 minutes, or until the mushrooms are tender and the filling is hot.

7. Remove the stuffed mushrooms from the oven and season with salt and pepper to taste.

8. Serve the quinoa stuffed portobello mushrooms warm, garnished with additional fresh basil if desired.

These vegetarian stuffed mushrooms make a delicious and healthy main dish or appetizer. The quinoa filling provides protein and fiber, while the feta cheese and fresh basil add tons of flavor. The portobello mushroom caps become tender and juicy in the oven.

42. Steamed Broccoli with Garlic

Ingredients:
- 1 lb broccoli florets
- 2 tablespoons olive oil
- 3 cloves garlic, minced
- 1/4 teaspoon red pepper flakes (optional)
- Salt and pepper to taste
- Lemon wedges for serving (optional)

Instructions:

1. Fill a medium saucepan with about 1 inch of water and bring it to a boil over high heat.

2. Place the broccoli florets in a steamer basket and carefully lower it into the saucepan. Cover the pot with a lid.

3. Steam the broccoli for 5-7 minutes, until it is tender but still crisp. The timing may vary depending on the size of your broccoli florets.

4. While the broccoli is steaming, heat the olive oil in a small skillet over medium heat. Add the minced garlic and sauté for 1-2 minutes, until fragrant and lightly golden.

5. Remove the steamed broccoli from the pot and transfer it to a serving bowl. Drizzle the garlic olive oil over the broccoli and toss to coat evenly.

6. If using, sprinkle the red pepper flakes over the broccoli. Season with salt and pepper to taste.

7. Serve the steamed broccoli with garlic immediately, with lemon wedges on the side if desired.

This simple preparation allows the fresh, natural flavor of the broccoli to shine, while the garlic adds a delicious savory note. The red pepper flakes provide a subtle heat.

Steamed broccoli with garlic makes a great side dish to accompany grilled or roasted meats, fish, or vegetarian main courses. Enjoy!

43. Lentil and Spinach Salad with Balsamic Dressing

Ingredients:
- 1 cup cooked lentils, cooled
- 5 oz baby spinach
- 1 cup cherry tomatoes, halved
- 1/2 cup crumbled feta cheese
- 1/4 cup sliced red onion
- 2 tablespoons chopped fresh parsley
- 2 tablespoons balsamic vinegar
- 1 tablespoon olive oil
- 1 teaspoon Dijon mustard
- 1 teaspoon honey
- Salt and pepper to taste

Instructions:

1. In a large salad bowl, combine the cooked and cooled lentils, baby spinach, halved cherry tomatoes, crumbled feta cheese, sliced red onion, and chopped fresh parsley.

2. In a small bowl, whisk together the balsamic vinegar, olive oil, Dijon mustard, and honey until emulsified. Season the dressing with salt and pepper to taste.

3. Drizzle the balsamic dressing over the lentil and spinach salad and toss gently to coat everything evenly.

4. Serve the lentil and spinach salad immediately, or refrigerate until ready to serve.

Tips:
- To cook the lentils, simmer 1/2 cup dry lentils in 1 1/2 cups of water or broth for 15-20 minutes until tender. Drain and cool before adding to the salad.
- For extra protein, you can add grilled chicken, shrimp, or hard-boiled eggs to the salad.
- Customize the salad by adding other vegetables like cucumber, bell pepper, or roasted beets.

This lentil and spinach salad is a nutritious and flavorful meal or side dish. The earthy lentils, fresh spinach, tangy feta, and balsamic dressing create a delicious balance of textures and flavors. Enjoy!

44. Lemon Herb Roasted Chicken

Ingredients:
- 1 (4-5 lb) whole chicken
- 2 lemons, halved
- 4 sprigs fresh thyme
- 4 sprigs fresh rosemary
- 4 cloves garlic, peeled and smashed
- 2 tablespoons olive oil
- 1 teaspoon salt
- 1/2 teaspoon black pepper

Instructions:

1. Preheat your oven to 425°F (220°C).

2. Pat the chicken dry with paper towels and place it in a large roasting pan or baking dish.

3. Stuff the cavity of the chicken with the halved lemons, sprigs of thyme and rosemary, and the smashed garlic cloves.

4. Drizzle the olive oil over the outside of the chicken and use your hands to rub it all over the skin. Season the chicken generously with salt and pepper.

5. Roast the chicken for 1 to 1 1/2 hours, or until the internal temperature reaches 165°F (75°C) when measured in the thickest part of the thigh. The juices should run clear when the chicken is pierced with a fork.

6. Remove the chicken from the oven and let it rest for 10-15 minutes before carving and serving.

7. Carve the chicken and serve it warm, drizzling any pan juices over the top. Garnish with the roasted lemon halves and fresh herb sprigs if desired.

The lemon, thyme, and rosemary infuse the chicken with bright, aromatic flavors as it roasts. The high heat helps create a crispy, golden-brown skin.

Serve the lemon herb roasted chicken with roasted vegetables, mashed potatoes, or a fresh salad for a complete and delicious meal. Enjoy!

45. Vegetable and Bean Chili

Ingredients:
- 2 tablespoons olive oil
- 1 onion, diced
- 3 cloves garlic, minced
- 1 red bell pepper, diced
- 1 zucchini, diced
- 1 (15 oz) can black beans, rinsed and drained
- 1 (15 oz) can kidney beans, rinsed and drained
- 1 (15 oz) can diced tomatoes
- 1 (6 oz) can tomato paste
- 2 tablespoons chili powder
- 1 teaspoon ground cumin
- 1 teaspoon dried oregano
- 1/2 teaspoon smoked paprika
- 1/4 teaspoon cayenne pepper (or to taste)
- Salt and pepper to taste
- Chopped cilantro for garnish (optional)

Instructions:

1. In a large pot or Dutch oven, heat the olive oil over medium heat. Add the diced onion and sauté for 5 minutes until translucent.

2. Add the minced garlic and sauté for 1 minute more, until fragrant.

3. Stir in the diced red bell pepper and zucchini. Cook for 5-7 minutes, until the vegetables start to soften.

4. Add the rinsed and drained black beans and kidney beans, diced tomatoes, tomato paste, chili powder, cumin, oregano, smoked paprika, and cayenne pepper.

5. Stir to combine all the ingredients and bring the chili to a simmer. Reduce the heat to medium-low.

6. Let the chili simmer for 20-25 minutes, stirring occasionally, until the vegetables are tender and the flavors have melded.

7. Season the chili with salt and pepper to taste.

8. Serve the vegetable and bean chili hot, garnished with chopped fresh cilantro if desired. Enjoy with cornbread, tortilla chips, or a side salad.

This hearty, vegetable-packed chili is a delicious meatless main dish. The combination of beans, bell pepper, zucchini, and warm spices creates a satisfying and flavorful chili. Adjust the amount of cayenne to control the heat level.

46. Spiced Roasted Carrots

Ingredients:
- 1 lb carrots, peeled and cut into 1-inch pieces
- 2 tablespoons olive oil
- 1 teaspoon ground cumin
- 1 teaspoon ground coriander
- 1/2 teaspoon smoked paprika
- 1/4 teaspoon cayenne pepper (or to taste)
- 1 teaspoon honey
- Salt and pepper to taste
- Chopped fresh parsley for garnish (optional)

Instructions:
1. Preheat your oven to 400°F (200°C). Line a baking sheet with parchment paper.

2. In a large bowl, toss the peeled and cut carrots with the olive oil, ground cumin, ground coriander, smoked paprika, and cayenne pepper.

3. Drizzle the honey over the carrots and season with salt and pepper. Toss to coat the carrots evenly.

4. Spread the seasoned carrots in a single layer on the prepared baking sheet.

5. Roast the carrots for 20-25 minutes, flipping them halfway through, until they are tender and lightly caramelized.

6. Remove the roasted carrots from the oven and transfer them to a serving dish.

7. Garnish the spiced roasted carrots with chopped fresh parsley, if desired.

Serve these flavorful roasted carrots as a side dish or enjoy them as a healthy snack. The combination of warm spices, honey, and high-heat roasting brings out the natural sweetness of the carrots.

You can adjust the amount of cayenne pepper to control the level of heat. For a milder version, you can omit the cayenne altogether.

47. Grilled Mahi Mahi with Mango Salsa

Ingredients:
For the Mango Salsa:
- 1 ripe mango, diced
- 1/2 red onion, finely chopped
- 1 jalapeño, seeded and finely chopped
- 1/4 cup chopped fresh cilantro
- 2 tablespoons lime juice
- 1/4 teaspoon salt

For the Grilled Mahi Mahi:
- 4 (6 oz) mahi mahi fillets
- 2 tablespoons olive oil
- 1 teaspoon chili powder
- 1/2 teaspoon garlic powder
- Salt and pepper to taste

Instructions:

1. Make the mango salsa: In a medium bowl, combine the diced mango, chopped red onion, jalapeño, cilantro, lime juice, and salt. Stir to mix well. Cover and refrigerate until ready to serve.

2. Prepare the mahi mahi: Pat the fish fillets dry with paper towels. Brush both sides of the fillets with the olive oil and season with the chili powder, garlic powder, salt, and pepper.

3. Preheat your grill or grill pan to medium-high heat.

4. Grill the mahi mahi fillets for 3-4 minutes per side, or until the fish flakes easily with a fork and reaches an internal temperature of 145°F (63°C).

5. Transfer the grilled mahi mahi fillets to a serving platter. Top each fillet with a generous spoonful of the chilled mango salsa.

6. Serve the grilled mahi mahi with mango salsa immediately, garnished with extra chopped cilantro if desired.

The sweet and tangy mango salsa complements the mild, flaky mahi mahi perfectly. The grilled fish and fresh salsa make for a light, healthy, and flavorful meal.

48. Caprese Salad with Balsamic Glaze

Ingredients:
- 8 oz fresh mozzarella cheese, sliced
- 2 large tomatoes, sliced
- 1/4 cup fresh basil leaves
- 2 tablespoons olive oil
- 2 tablespoons balsamic vinegar
- 1 tablespoon balsamic glaze (or reduced balsamic vinegar)
- Salt and pepper to taste

Instructions:
1. Arrange the sliced mozzarella cheese and tomatoes on a serving platter or plate, alternating the layers.

2. Scatter the fresh basil leaves over the top of the cheese and tomatoes.

3. In a small bowl, whisk together the olive oil and balsamic vinegar. Drizzle this dressing over the Caprese salad.

4. Drizzle the balsamic glaze over the top of the salad in a zig-zag pattern.

5. Season the Caprese salad with salt and freshly ground black pepper to taste.

6. Let the salad sit for 5-10 minutes to allow the flavors to meld together.

7. Serve the Caprese salad immediately, or chill it in the refrigerator until ready to serve.

Tips:
- Use the freshest, ripest tomatoes and high-quality mozzarella cheese for the best flavor.
- You can make your own balsamic glaze by simmering balsamic vinegar until it reduces by half and becomes thicker.
- For added flavor, you can sprinkle a bit of dried oregano or crushed red pepper flakes over the salad.

This simple Caprese salad showcases the classic combination of juicy tomatoes, creamy mozzarella, and fragrant basil, all drizzled with a sweet balsamic glaze. It's a perfect light and refreshing summer dish

49. Eggplant and Tomato Bake

Ingredients:
- 1 medium eggplant, cut into 1/2-inch thick slices
- 2 tablespoons olive oil, plus more for drizzling
- 1 onion, diced
- 3 cloves garlic, minced
- 1 (14.5 oz) can diced tomatoes
- 1 teaspoon dried oregano
- 1/2 teaspoon dried basil
- Salt and pepper to taste
- 1 cup shredded mozzarella cheese
- 1/4 cup grated Parmesan cheese

Instructions:

1. Preheat your oven to 375°F (190°C). Grease a 9x13 inch baking dish.

2. Arrange the eggplant slices in a single layer on a baking sheet. Drizzle both sides with olive oil and season with salt and pepper.

3. Roast the eggplant slices for 15-20 minutes, flipping halfway, until they are tender and lightly browned. Remove from the oven and set aside.

4. In a skillet, heat 2 tablespoons of olive oil over medium heat. Add the diced onion and sauté for 5 minutes until translucent.

5. Add the minced garlic and cook for 1 minute more, until fragrant.

6. Stir in the diced tomatoes, dried oregano, and dried basil. Season with salt and pepper to taste.

7. Arrange the roasted eggplant slices in the prepared baking dish. Pour the tomato mixture over the top, spreading it evenly.

8. Sprinkle the shredded mozzarella cheese and grated Parmesan cheese over the top.

9. Bake the eggplant and tomato bake for 25-30 minutes, until the cheese is melted and bubbly. Remove the bake from the oven and let it cool for 5 minutes before serving.

Serve the eggplant and tomato bake warm, garnished with extra fresh basil if desired. This makes a great vegetarian main dish or side.

50. Thai Vegetable and Tofu Stir-Fry

Ingredients:
- 1 block (14 oz) extra-firm tofu, cubed
- 2 tablespoons vegetable oil
- 1 red bell pepper, sliced
- 1 cup broccoli florets
- 1 cup sliced mushrooms
- 1 cup snow peas or snap peas
- 3 cloves garlic, minced
- 1 tablespoon grated fresh ginger
- 2 tablespoons soy sauce
- 1 tablespoon fish sauce
- 1 tablespoon brown sugar
- 1 teaspoon red curry paste (or more to taste)
- 1/4 cup chopped fresh cilantro
- Cooked jasmine rice, for serving

Instructions:
1. Press the tofu block between paper towels or a clean kitchen towel to remove excess moisture. Cut the tofu into 1-inch cubes.

2. Heat the vegetable oil in a large skillet or wok over medium-high heat. Add the cubed tofu and cook, stirring occasionally, until lightly browned on all sides, about 5-7 minutes. Transfer the tofu to a plate.

3. In the same skillet, add the sliced red bell pepper, broccoli florets, sliced mushrooms, and snow peas. Stir-fry for 3-4 minutes until the vegetables are crisp-tender.

4. Add the minced garlic and grated ginger to the skillet. Cook for 1 minute, until fragrant.

5. Stir in the soy sauce, fish sauce, brown sugar, and red curry paste. Bring the mixture to a simmer.

6. Add the cooked tofu back to the skillet and toss everything together to coat the tofu and vegetables in the sauce.

7. Remove the skillet from the heat and stir in the chopped fresh cilantro. Serve the Thai vegetable and tofu stir-fry immediately over steamed jasmine rice.

This colorful and flavorful stir-fry is packed with fresh vegetables and protein-rich tofu. The Thai-inspired sauce with soy, fish sauce, and red curry paste adds a delicious savory and slightly spicy element

51. Cabbage and Apple Slaw

Ingredients:
- 1/2 head of green cabbage, thinly sliced
- 2 medium apples, cored and thinly sliced (you can use your favorite variety, such as Granny Smith or Honeycrisp)
- 1/4 cup chopped fresh parsley
- 1/4 cup mayonnaise
- 2 tablespoons apple cider vinegar
- 1 tablespoon honey or maple syrup
- Salt and pepper to taste
- Optional: 1/4 cup chopped nuts (such as walnuts or pecans) for added crunch

Instructions:

1. In a large mixing bowl, combine the sliced cabbage, sliced apples, and chopped parsley.

2. In a small bowl, whisk together the mayonnaise, apple cider vinegar, honey or maple syrup, salt, and pepper until well combined.

3. Pour the dressing over the cabbage, apples, and parsley. Toss everything together until the cabbage and apples are evenly coated with the dressing.

4. If using chopped nuts, sprinkle them over the slaw and toss to combine.

5. Taste and adjust seasoning if necessary. You can add more salt, pepper, or honey/maple syrup according to your preference.

6. Cover the bowl and refrigerate the slaw for at least 30 minutes to allow the flavors to meld together.

7. Serve chilled as a side dish or as a topping for sandwiches, tacos, or burgers. Enjoy your refreshing Cabbage and Apple Slaw!

52. Roasted Brussels Sprouts with Bacon

Ingredients:
- 1 lb Brussels sprouts, trimmed and halved
- 4-6 slices of bacon, chopped into small pieces
- 2 tablespoons olive oil
- Salt and pepper to taste
- Optional: grated Parmesan cheese for serving

Instructions:
1. Preheat your oven to 400°F (200°C).

2. In a large mixing bowl, toss the Brussels sprouts with olive oil until they are evenly coated. Season with salt and pepper to taste.

3. Spread the Brussels sprouts out in a single layer on a baking sheet lined with parchment paper or aluminum foil.

4. Scatter the chopped bacon pieces over the Brussels sprouts.

5. Roast in the preheated oven for about 20-25 minutes, or until the Brussels sprouts are tender and caramelized, and the bacon is crispy. Stir the Brussels sprouts and bacon halfway through the cooking time to ensure even roasting.

6. Once done, remove the baking sheet from the oven and transfer the roasted Brussels sprouts and bacon to a serving dish.

7. If desired, sprinkle some grated Parmesan cheese over the top before serving.

8. Serve hot as a delicious side dish alongside your favorite main course. Enjoy your Roasted Brussels Sprouts with Bacon!

53. Stuffed Acorn Squash with Quinoa and Cranberries

Ingredients:
- 2 acorn squash, halved and seeds removed
- 1 cup quinoa, rinsed
- 2 cups vegetable broth or water
- 1/2 cup dried cranberries
- 1/2 cup chopped pecans or walnuts
- 1 small onion, finely chopped
- 2 cloves garlic, minced
- 2 tablespoons olive oil
- 1 teaspoon dried thyme
- Salt and pepper to taste
- Optional: crumbled feta or goat cheese for serving
- Fresh parsley or thyme for garnish

Instructions:
1. Preheat your oven to 400°F (200°C).

2. Place the acorn squash halves cut side down on a baking sheet lined with parchment paper. Bake in the preheated oven for about 30-35 minutes, or until the squash is tender when pierced with a fork.

3. While the squash is baking, prepare the quinoa. In a medium saucepan, bring the vegetable broth or water to a boil. Add the quinoa, reduce the heat to low, cover, and simmer for about 15 minutes, or until the quinoa is cooked and the liquid is absorbed. Remove from heat and fluff with a fork.

4. In a skillet, heat the olive oil over medium heat. Add the chopped onion and cook until softened, about 3-4 minutes. Add the minced garlic and cook for an additional 1-2 minutes, until fragrant.

5. Add the cooked quinoa, dried cranberries, chopped nuts, dried thyme, salt, and pepper to the skillet with the onions and garlic. Stir to combine and cook for another 2-3 minutes to allow the flavors to meld together.

6. Once the squash halves are tender, remove them from the oven and carefully flip them over using tongs or a spatula.

7. Stuff each squash half with the quinoa mixture, pressing down gently to pack it in. If desired, sprinkle crumbled feta or goat cheese over the top of each stuffed squash half.

8. Return the stuffed squash to the oven and bake for an additional 10-15 minutes, or until heated through and the tops are lightly golden.

9. Remove from the oven and garnish with fresh parsley or thyme before serving. Serve hot as a delicious and nutritious vegetarian main dish. Enjoy your Stuffed Acorn Squash with Quinoa and Cranberries!

54. Lemon Garlic Roasted Shrimp

Ingredients:
- 1 lb large shrimp, peeled and deveined
- 3 cloves garlic, minced
- Zest of 1 lemon
- Juice of 1 lemon
- 2 tablespoons olive oil
- 1 teaspoon dried oregano
- 1/2 teaspoon paprika
- Salt and pepper to taste
- Fresh parsley, chopped, for garnish

Instructions:
1. Preheat your oven to 400°F (200°C).

2. In a mixing bowl, combine the minced garlic, lemon zest, lemon juice, olive oil, dried oregano, paprika, salt, and pepper.

3. Add the peeled and deveined shrimp to the bowl and toss to coat them evenly with the lemon garlic mixture.

4. Arrange the shrimp in a single layer on a baking sheet lined with parchment paper or aluminum foil.

5. Roast the shrimp in the preheated oven for about 8-10 minutes, or until they are pink and opaque.

6. Once done, remove the shrimp from the oven and garnish with chopped fresh parsley.

7. Serve the Lemon Garlic Roasted Shrimp hot as a main dish with your favorite sides, such as rice, pasta, or a salad.

8. Enjoy your flavorful and easy-to-make Lemon Garlic Roasted Shrimp!

55. Edamame and Carrot Salad

Ingredients:
- 2 cups shelled edamame (frozen or fresh)
- 2 cups shredded carrots
- 1/4 cup chopped fresh cilantro or parsley
- 2 tablespoons sesame seeds
- 2 tablespoons rice vinegar
- 1 tablespoon soy sauce
- 1 tablespoon honey or maple syrup
- 1 tablespoon sesame oil
- 1 clove garlic, minced
- Salt and pepper to taste

Instructions:
1. If using frozen edamame, cook them according to the package instructions. If using fresh edamame, blanch them in boiling water for 3-4 minutes, then drain and rinse them under cold water.

2. In a large mixing bowl, combine the cooked edamame, shredded carrots, chopped cilantro or parsley, and sesame seeds.

3. In a small bowl, whisk together the rice vinegar, soy sauce, honey or maple syrup, sesame oil, minced garlic, salt, and pepper to make the dressing.

4. Pour the dressing over the edamame and carrot mixture, and toss until everything is evenly coated.

5. Taste and adjust the seasoning if necessary.

6. Cover the bowl and refrigerate the salad for at least 30 minutes to allow the flavors to meld together.

7. Before serving, give the salad a final toss and garnish with additional sesame seeds and chopped cilantro or parsley if desired.

8. Serve the Edamame and Carrot Salad chilled as a side dish or light meal.

9. Enjoy the vibrant colors and fresh flavors of this delicious salad!

56. Sesame Ginger Tofu Stir-Fry

Ingredients:

- 14 oz (400g) firm tofu, pressed and cubed
- 2 tablespoons soy sauce
- 2 tablespoons sesame oil
- 2 tablespoons rice vinegar
- 1 tablespoon honey or maple syrup
- 1 tablespoon grated fresh ginger
- 2 cloves garlic, minced
- 1 tablespoon cornstarch
- 2 tablespoons vegetable oil, for cooking
- 1 bell pepper, sliced
- 1 cup broccoli florets
- 1 carrot, julienned
- 2 green onions, sliced
- Sesame seeds for garnish
- Cooked rice or noodles, for serving

Instructions:

1. In a mixing bowl, combine the soy sauce, sesame oil, rice vinegar, honey or maple syrup, grated ginger, minced garlic, and cornstarch. Whisk until the cornstarch is dissolved and the sauce is well combined.

2. Add the cubed tofu to the bowl and gently toss to coat it in the marinade. Let it marinate for at least 15-20 minutes.

3. Heat the vegetable oil in a large skillet or wok over medium-high heat. Add the marinated tofu cubes (reserving any excess marinade) and cook until golden brown and crispy on all sides, about 5-7 minutes. Remove the tofu from the skillet and set it aside.

4. In the same skillet, add a little more oil if needed. Add the sliced bell pepper, broccoli florets, and julienned carrot. Stir-fry for about 3-4 minutes, or until the vegetables are tender-crisp.

5. Return the cooked tofu to the skillet, along with any reserved marinade. Stir everything together and cook for an additional 2-3 minutes, or until the sauce has thickened slightly and everything is heated through.

6. Taste and adjust the seasoning if necessary. You can add more soy sauce or honey/maple syrup according to your taste.

7. Remove the skillet from the heat and sprinkle sliced green onions and sesame seeds over the top.

8. Serve the Sesame Ginger Tofu Stir-Fry hot over cooked rice or noodles.

9. Enjoy the delicious combination of flavors and textures in this satisfying stir-fry dish!

57. Roasted Beet and Goat Cheese Salad

Ingredients:
- 3 medium beets, washed and trimmed
- 4 cups mixed greens (such as arugula, spinach, or baby kale)
- 1/4 cup crumbled goat cheese
- 1/4 cup chopped walnuts or pecans, toasted
- 2 tablespoons balsamic vinegar
- 2 tablespoons extra virgin olive oil
- Salt and pepper to taste

Instructions:
1. Preheat your oven to 400°F (200°C).

2. Wrap each beet individually in aluminum foil and place them on a baking sheet. Roast in the preheated oven for about 45-60 minutes, or until the beets are tender when pierced with a fork. Let them cool slightly.

3. Once the beets are cool enough to handle, peel off the skins using your fingers or a small knife. Cut the beets into bite-sized wedges or slices.

4. In a small bowl, whisk together the balsamic vinegar, extra virgin olive oil, salt, and pepper to make the dressing.

5. Place the mixed greens in a large salad bowl. Add the roasted beet slices on top.

6. Drizzle the dressing over the salad and gently toss everything together until the greens are evenly coated.

7. Sprinkle the crumbled goat cheese and toasted nuts over the top of the salad.

8. Serve the Roasted Beet and Goat Cheese Salad immediately as a side dish or light meal.

9. Enjoy the vibrant colors and delicious flavors of this simple and elegant salad!

58. Greek Yogurt Chicken Salad

Ingredients:
- 2 cups cooked chicken breast, shredded or diced
- 1/2 cup Greek yogurt (plain)
- 1/4 cup diced celery
- 1/4 cup diced red onion
- 1/4 cup halved grapes
- 1/4 cup chopped walnuts or pecans
- 1 tablespoon lemon juice
- 1 tablespoon Dijon mustard
- 1 tablespoon honey or maple syrup
- Salt and pepper to taste
- Optional: chopped fresh herbs such as parsley or dill

 Instructions:
1. In a large mixing bowl, combine the cooked chicken breast, diced celery, diced red onion, halved grapes, and chopped nuts.

2. In a separate small bowl, whisk together the Greek yogurt, lemon juice, Dijon mustard, honey or maple syrup, salt, and pepper until well combined.

3. Pour the Greek yogurt dressing over the chicken mixture in the large bowl.

4. Gently toss everything together until the chicken and other ingredients are evenly coated with the dressing.

5. Taste and adjust the seasoning if necessary. You can add more salt, pepper, lemon juice, or honey/maple syrup according to your preference.

6. If using, sprinkle chopped fresh herbs over the top of the chicken salad for added flavor and freshness.

7. Cover the bowl and refrigerate the chicken salad for at least 30 minutes to allow the flavors to meld together.

8. Serve the Greek Yogurt Chicken Salad chilled on its own, on a bed of lettuce, or as a sandwich filling.

9. Enjoy this lighter and protein-packed version of chicken salad!

59. Balsamic Glazed Roasted Vegetables

Ingredients:
- 4 cups mixed vegetables, chopped (such as bell peppers, zucchini, carrots, cherry tomatoes, red onion, mushrooms, etc.)
- 2 tablespoons olive oil
- 2 tablespoons balsamic vinegar
- 2 cloves garlic, minced
- 1 tablespoon honey or maple syrup
- 1 teaspoon dried Italian herbs (such as oregano, thyme, or rosemary)
- Salt and pepper to taste
- Fresh parsley, chopped, for garnish (optional)

Instructions:
1. Preheat your oven to 425°F (220°C).

2. In a large mixing bowl, combine the chopped vegetables with olive oil, balsamic vinegar, minced garlic, honey or maple syrup, dried Italian herbs, salt, and pepper. Toss until the vegetables are evenly coated.

3. Spread the vegetables out in a single layer on a large baking sheet lined with parchment paper or aluminum foil.

4. Roast the vegetables in the preheated oven for about 20-25 minutes, or until they are tender and caramelized, stirring halfway through the cooking time for even roasting.

5. Once the vegetables are done, remove them from the oven and transfer them to a serving dish.

6. If desired, sprinkle chopped fresh parsley over the top for added freshness and flavor.

7. Serve the Balsamic Glazed Roasted Vegetables hot as a side dish alongside your favorite main course.

8. Enjoy the delicious combination of flavors and textures in this vibrant dish!

60. Spinach and Mushroom Frittata

Ingredients:
- 8 large eggs
- 1/4 cup milk or heavy cream
- 1 tablespoon olive oil
- 1 small onion, finely chopped
- 2 cloves garlic, minced
- 8 oz (225g) mushrooms, sliced
- 2 cups fresh spinach leaves
- 1/2 cup shredded cheese (such as cheddar, mozzarella, or feta)
- Salt and pepper to taste
- Optional: chopped fresh herbs (such as parsley or chives) for garnish

Instructions:
1. Preheat your oven to 350°F (175°C).

2. In a mixing bowl, whisk together the eggs, milk or heavy cream, salt, and pepper until well combined. Set aside.

3. Heat the olive oil in a large oven-safe skillet over medium heat. Add the chopped onion and cook until softened, about 3-4 minutes.

4. Add the minced garlic and sliced mushrooms to the skillet. Cook for another 5-6 minutes, or until the mushrooms are tender and any liquid has evaporated.

5. Add the fresh spinach leaves to the skillet and cook for 1-2 minutes, or until wilted.

6. Pour the egg mixture evenly over the vegetables in the skillet. Let it cook undisturbed for about 2 minutes, or until the edges start to set.

7. Sprinkle the shredded cheese evenly over the top of the frittata.

8. Transfer the skillet to the preheated oven and bake for 12-15 minutes, or until the frittata is set in the center and the top is golden brown.

9. Once done, remove the skillet from the oven and let the frittata cool slightly for a few minutes.

10. Carefully slide a spatula around the edges of the skillet to loosen the frittata. Slide it onto a serving plate or cutting board. Slice the frittata into wedges and garnish with chopped fresh herbs if desired.

11. Serve the Spinach and Mushroom Frittata warm or at room temperature as a delicious and satisfying meal. Enjoy the wonderful flavors and textures of this easy-to-make frittata!

61. Turmeric Roasted Cauliflower

Ingredients:
- 1 head cauliflower, cut into florets
- 2 tablespoons olive oil
- 1 teaspoon ground turmeric
- 1/2 teaspoon ground cumin
- 1/2 teaspoon ground paprika
- 1/4 teaspoon ground coriander
- Salt and pepper to taste
- Fresh cilantro or parsley for garnish (optional)
- Lemon wedges for serving (optional)

Instructions:
1. Preheat your oven to 425°F (220°C).

2. In a large mixing bowl, combine the cauliflower florets with olive oil, ground turmeric, ground cumin, ground paprika, ground coriander, salt, and pepper. Toss until the cauliflower is evenly coated with the spices and oil.

3. Spread the seasoned cauliflower florets out in a single layer on a large baking sheet lined with parchment paper or aluminum foil.

4. Roast the cauliflower in the preheated oven for about 25-30 minutes, or until it is tender and golden brown, stirring halfway through the cooking time for even roasting.

5. Once done, remove the cauliflower from the oven and transfer it to a serving dish.

6. If desired, garnish the Turmeric Roasted Cauliflower with fresh cilantro or parsley before serving.

7. Serve hot as a flavorful side dish alongside your favorite main course.

8. Optionally, squeeze some fresh lemon juice over the roasted cauliflower for a bright and refreshing flavor.

9. Enjoy the delicious and aromatic Turmeric Roasted Cauliflower as part of your meal!

62. Mediterranean Quinoa Salad

Ingredients:
- 1 cup quinoa, rinsed
- 2 cups water or vegetable broth
- 1 cup cherry tomatoes, halved
- 1 cucumber, diced
- 1/2 red onion, finely chopped
- 1/2 cup Kalamata olives, sliced
- 1/2 cup crumbled feta cheese
- 1/4 cup chopped fresh parsley
- 1/4 cup chopped fresh mint leaves
- 1/4 cup extra virgin olive oil
- 2 tablespoons lemon juice
- 2 cloves garlic, minced
- 1 teaspoon dried oregano
- Salt and pepper to taste

Instructions:
1. In a medium saucepan, combine the quinoa and water or vegetable broth. Bring to a boil, then reduce the heat to low, cover, and simmer for about 15 minutes, or until the quinoa is cooked and the liquid is absorbed. Remove from heat and let it cool slightly.

2. In a large mixing bowl, combine the cooked quinoa, cherry tomatoes, cucumber, red onion, Kalamata olives, crumbled feta cheese, chopped parsley, and chopped mint leaves.

3. In a small bowl, whisk together the extra virgin olive oil, lemon juice, minced garlic, dried oregano, salt, and pepper to make the dressing.

4. Pour the dressing over the quinoa salad and toss until everything is evenly coated.

5. Taste and adjust the seasoning if necessary. You can add more salt, pepper, or lemon juice according to your preference.

6. Cover the bowl and refrigerate the Mediterranean Quinoa Salad for at least 30 minutes to allow the flavors to meld together.

7. Before serving, give the salad a final toss and garnish with additional fresh parsley or mint leaves if desired.

8. Serve the salad chilled as a refreshing side dish or light meal. Enjoy the vibrant colors and delicious flavors of this Mediterranean-inspired quinoa salad!

63. Honey Mustard Glazed Salmon

Ingredients:
- 4 salmon fillets, skin-on or skinless
- 2 tablespoons honey
- 2 tablespoons Dijon mustard
- 1 tablespoon whole grain mustard
- 1 tablespoon soy sauce
- 2 cloves garlic, minced
- 1 tablespoon olive oil
- Salt and pepper to taste
- Fresh parsley, chopped, for garnish (optional)
- Lemon wedges for serving (optional)

Instructions:
1. Preheat your oven to 400°F (200°C).

2. In a small bowl, whisk together the honey, Dijon mustard, whole grain mustard, soy sauce, minced garlic, olive oil, salt, and pepper to make the glaze.

3. Place the salmon fillets on a baking sheet lined with parchment paper or aluminum foil. If the salmon has skin, place it skin-side down.

4. Brush the honey mustard glaze evenly over the top of each salmon fillet, coating them generously.

5. Bake the salmon in the preheated oven for about 12-15 minutes, or until the salmon is cooked through and flakes easily with a fork.

6. Once done, remove the salmon from the oven and let it rest for a few minutes.

7. If desired, garnish the Honey Mustard Glazed Salmon with chopped fresh parsley and serve with lemon wedges on the side for squeezing over the salmon before eating.

8. Serve the salmon hot as a delicious and nutritious main dish.

9. Enjoy the sweet and tangy flavors of this Honey Mustard Glazed Salmon!

64. Kale and Avocado Salad with Lemon Dressing

Ingredients:
- 4 cups kale leaves, stems removed and thinly sliced
- 1 ripe avocado, diced
- 1/4 cup sliced red onion
- 1/4 cup cherry tomatoes, halved
- 1/4 cup toasted pumpkin seeds or sunflower seeds
- 1/4 cup crumbled feta cheese or goat cheese (optional)
- 2 tablespoons extra virgin olive oil
- 2 tablespoons lemon juice
- 1 clove garlic, minced
- 1 teaspoon honey or maple syrup
- Salt and pepper to taste

Instructions:
1. In a large mixing bowl, combine the thinly sliced kale leaves, diced avocado, sliced red onion, halved cherry tomatoes, and toasted pumpkin seeds.

2. In a small bowl, whisk together the extra virgin olive oil, lemon juice, minced garlic, honey or maple syrup, salt, and pepper to make the dressing.

3. Pour the dressing over the kale and avocado mixture in the large bowl.

4. Using clean hands, gently massage the dressing into the kale leaves for a minute or two. This will help soften the kale and infuse it with flavor.

5. Taste and adjust the seasoning if necessary.

6. If using, sprinkle crumbled feta cheese or goat cheese over the top of the salad for added creaminess and flavor.

7. Serve the Kale and Avocado Salad immediately as a side dish or light meal.

8. Enjoy the fresh and vibrant flavors of this nutritious salad!

Feel free to customize this salad by adding other ingredients such as sliced cucumber, shredded carrots, or cooked grains like quinoa or bulgur.

65. Spaghetti Squash Pad Thai

Ingredients:
- 1 medium spaghetti squash
- 2 tablespoons vegetable oil
- 2 cloves garlic, minced
- 1 small onion, thinly sliced
- 1 red bell pepper, thinly sliced
- 2 carrots, julienned
- 1 cup bean sprouts
- 2 green onions, sliced
- 1/4 cup chopped peanuts, for garnish
- Lime wedges, for serving

For the sauce:
- 1/4 cup soy sauce
- 2 tablespoons fish sauce (optional, for a more authentic flavor)
- 2 tablespoons rice vinegar
- 1 tablespoon brown sugar or honey
- 1 tablespoon Sriracha sauce (adjust to taste)
- Juice of 1 lime

Optional protein:
- 2 eggs, lightly beaten
- 8 oz (225g) cooked shrimp, chicken, or tofu

Instructions:
1. Preheat your oven to 400°F (200°C).

2. Cut the spaghetti squash in half lengthwise and scoop out the seeds. Place the squash halves cut side down on a baking sheet lined with parchment paper.

3. Roast the squash in the preheated oven for about 40-45 minutes, or until the flesh is tender and can be easily shredded into strands with a fork. Remove from the oven and let it cool slightly.

4. While the squash is roasting, prepare the sauce by whisking together the soy sauce, fish sauce (if using), rice vinegar, brown sugar or honey, Sriracha sauce, and lime juice in a small bowl. Set aside.

5. In a large skillet or wok, heat the vegetable oil over medium-high heat. Add the minced garlic and sliced onion, and cook for 2-3 minutes until softened and fragrant. Add the sliced bell pepper and julienned carrots to the skillet, and stir-fry for another 3-4 minutes until the vegetables are tender-crisp.

7. If using, push the vegetables to one side of the skillet and add the beaten eggs to the empty side. Cook, stirring occasionally, until scrambled and cooked through.

8. Once the spaghetti squash is cool enough to handle, use a fork to scrape the flesh into strands. Add the spaghetti squash strands to the skillet along with the bean sprouts and sliced green onions.

9. Pour the prepared sauce over the squash and vegetables in the skillet. Toss everything together until well combined and heated through. If using, add the cooked shrimp, chicken, or tofu to the skillet and toss to combine with the squash and vegetables

66. Garlic Herb Roasted Potatoes

Ingredients:
- 2 lbs (about 900g) baby potatoes, halved or quartered if large
- 3 tablespoons olive oil
- 4 cloves garlic, minced
- 1 teaspoon dried thyme
- 1 teaspoon dried rosemary
- 1 teaspoon dried oregano
- Salt and pepper to taste
- Fresh parsley, chopped, for garnish (optional)

Instructions:
1. Preheat your oven to 425°F (220°C).

2. In a large mixing bowl, combine the halved or quartered baby potatoes with olive oil, minced garlic, dried thyme, dried rosemary, dried oregano, salt, and pepper. Toss until the potatoes are evenly coated with the herb mixture.

3. Spread the seasoned potatoes out in a single layer on a large baking sheet lined with parchment paper or aluminum foil.

4. Roast the potatoes in the preheated oven for about 30-35 minutes, or until they are golden brown and crispy on the outside, and tender on the inside. Stir or shake the pan halfway through the cooking time for even roasting.

5. Once done, remove the roasted potatoes from the oven and transfer them to a serving dish.

6. If desired, sprinkle chopped fresh parsley over the top for added freshness and flavor.

7. Serve the Garlic Herb Roasted Potatoes hot as a delicious side dish alongside your favorite main course.

8. Enjoy the wonderful aroma and comforting flavors of these roasted potatoes!

67. Seared Tuna Salad with Sesame Dressing

Ingredients:
For the seared tuna:
- 2 tuna steaks, about 6 oz (170g) each
- 1 tablespoon soy sauce
- 1 tablespoon sesame oil
- 1 teaspoon grated fresh ginger
- 1 clove garlic, minced
- Salt and pepper to taste
- 1 tablespoon vegetable oil (for searing)

For the sesame dressing:
- 3 tablespoons soy sauce
- 2 tablespoons rice vinegar
- 1 tablespoon sesame oil
- 1 tablespoon honey or maple syrup
- 1 teaspoon grated fresh ginger
- 1 clove garlic, minced

For the salad:
- 6 cups mixed salad greens
(such as lettuce, spinach,
arugula, or kale)
- 1 cucumber, thinly sliced
- 1 carrot, julienned
- 1 bell pepper, thinly sliced
- 1 avocado, sliced
- 2 green onions, sliced
- Sesame seeds for garnish

Instructions:

1. In a shallow dish, combine the soy sauce, sesame oil, grated ginger, minced garlic, salt, and pepper. Place the tuna steaks in the marinade, turning to coat both sides. Let them marinate for about 15-30 minutes.

2. While the tuna is marinating, prepare the salad ingredients. In a large bowl, combine the mixed salad greens, thinly sliced cucumber, julienned carrot, thinly sliced bell pepper, sliced avocado, and sliced green onions. Toss to combine.

3. In a small bowl, whisk together the ingredients for the sesame dressing: soy sauce, rice vinegar, sesame oil, honey or maple syrup, grated ginger, and minced garlic. Set aside.

4. Heat the vegetable oil in a skillet or grill pan over medium-high heat. Once hot, add the marinated tuna steaks and sear for about 1-2 minutes on each side, depending on the thickness of the steaks and your desired level of doneness. For rare tuna, sear for about 1 minute on each side. Remove from heat and let them rest for a few minutes.

5. Slice the seared tuna steaks thinly against the grain. To assemble the salad, divide the mixed greens and vegetables among serving plates. Arrange the sliced seared tuna on top.

6. Drizzle the sesame dressing over the salad. Sprinkle sesame seeds over the top for garnish. Serve the Seared Tuna Salad with Sesame Dressing immediately, and enjoy the delicious combination of flavors and textures!

68. Broccoli and Cauliflower Gratin

Ingredients:
- 1 head cauliflower, cut into florets
- 1 head broccoli, cut into florets
- 3 tablespoons butter
- 3 tablespoons all-purpose flour
- 2 cups milk
- 1 cup shredded cheddar cheese
- 1/4 cup grated Parmesan cheese
- 1/2 teaspoon garlic powder
- Salt and pepper to taste
- 1/2 cup breadcrumbs (optional, for topping)
- Fresh parsley, chopped, for garnish (optional)

Instructions:
1. Preheat your oven to 375°F (190°C). Lightly grease a baking dish with butter or cooking spray.

2. Bring a large pot of salted water to a boil. Add the cauliflower and broccoli florets and blanch them for about 3-4 minutes, or until slightly tender. Drain and set aside.

3. In a saucepan, melt the butter over medium heat. Add the flour and cook, stirring constantly, for about 1-2 minutes to make a roux.

4. Gradually whisk in the milk, stirring constantly to prevent lumps from forming. Cook the sauce until it thickens and bubbles, about 3-4 minutes.

5. Remove the saucepan from the heat and stir in the shredded cheddar cheese and grated Parmesan cheese until melted and smooth. Season with garlic powder, salt, and pepper to taste.

6. Add the blanched cauliflower and broccoli florets to the cheese sauce, stirring gently to coat them evenly.

7. Transfer the mixture to the prepared baking dish, spreading it out into an even layer. If desired, sprinkle breadcrumbs over the top of the gratin for added crunch and texture.

8. Bake the Broccoli and Cauliflower Gratin in the preheated oven for about 25-30 minutes, or until bubbly and golden brown on top.

9. Once done, remove the gratin from the oven and let it cool slightly before serving. Garnish with chopped fresh parsley if desired, and serve hot as a delicious side dish. Enjoy the creamy and cheesy goodness of this Broccoli and Cauliflower Gratin!

69. Beet and Orange Salad with Goat Cheese

Ingredients:
- 3 medium beets, cooked, peeled, and sliced
- 2 oranges, peeled and sliced
- 2 cups mixed salad greens (such as arugula, spinach, or mixed greens)
- 1/4 cup crumbled goat cheese
- 2 tablespoons chopped walnuts or pecans, toasted (optional)
- 2 tablespoons extra virgin olive oil
- 1 tablespoon balsamic vinegar
- 1 teaspoon honey or maple syrup
- Salt and pepper to taste

Instructions:
1. If you haven't cooked the beets yet, you can roast them in the oven until tender, then let them cool before peeling and slicing.

2. In a small bowl, whisk together the extra virgin olive oil, balsamic vinegar, honey or maple syrup, salt, and pepper to make the dressing. Set aside.

3. Arrange the sliced beets and oranges on a serving platter or individual plates, alternating them for a visually appealing presentation.

4. Place the mixed salad greens on top of the beets and oranges.

5. Drizzle the dressing over the salad, ensuring that everything is evenly coated.

6. Sprinkle crumbled goat cheese and chopped toasted nuts over the top of the salad.

7. Serve the Beet and Orange Salad with Goat Cheese immediately as a refreshing and nutritious appetizer or side dish.

8. Enjoy the delightful combination of flavors and textures in this vibrant salad!

70. Grilled Vegetable and Hummus Wrap

Ingredients:
- 1 large whole wheat or spinach tortilla wrap
- 1/4 cup hummus (store-bought or homemade)
- 1/2 cup mixed grilled vegetables (such as bell peppers, zucchini, eggplant, onions, mushrooms, etc.), sliced
- 1/4 cup baby spinach leaves
- 2 tablespoons crumbled feta cheese (optional)
- 1 tablespoon chopped fresh herbs (such as parsley or basil)
- Salt and pepper to taste
- Olive oil for grilling

Instructions:
1. Preheat a grill or grill pan over medium-high heat.

2. Brush the sliced mixed vegetables with olive oil and season with salt and pepper to taste.

3. Grill the vegetables for about 3-4 minutes on each side, or until they are tender and have nice grill marks. Remove from the grill and set aside.

4. Warm the tortilla wrap slightly in the microwave or on a skillet to make it more pliable.

5. Spread the hummus evenly over the center of the tortilla wrap, leaving a border around the edges.

6. Layer the grilled vegetables over the hummus.

7. Top the vegetables with baby spinach leaves, crumbled feta cheese (if using), and chopped fresh herbs.

8. Fold the sides of the tortilla inward, then roll it up tightly from the bottom to form a wrap.

9. Cut the wrap in half diagonally, if desired, and serve immediately.

10. Enjoy your Grilled Vegetable and Hummus Wrap as a delicious and nutritious meal!

Feel free to customize the wrap with your favorite grilled vegetables, add avocado slices, or drizzle with a balsamic glaze for extra flavor.

71. Lemon Herb Baked Tilapia

Ingredients:
- 4 tilapia fillets
- 2 tablespoons olive oil
- 2 tablespoons lemon juice
- 2 cloves garlic, minced
- 1 teaspoon dried thyme
- 1 teaspoon dried rosemary
- 1 teaspoon dried oregano
- Salt and pepper to taste
- Lemon slices for garnish
- Fresh parsley, chopped, for garnish

Instructions:
1. Preheat your oven to 400°F (200°C). Lightly grease a baking dish with olive oil or cooking spray.

2. Rinse the tilapia fillets under cold water and pat them dry with paper towels. Place them in the prepared baking dish.

3. In a small bowl, whisk together the olive oil, lemon juice, minced garlic, dried thyme, dried rosemary, dried oregano, salt, and pepper.

4. Pour the lemon herb marinade over the tilapia fillets, coating them evenly. You can use a brush or your hands to make sure the fillets are well coated.

5. Place a few lemon slices on top of each tilapia fillet for extra flavor and presentation.

6. Bake the tilapia in the preheated oven for about 12-15 minutes, or until the fish is opaque and flakes easily with a fork.

7. Once done, remove the tilapia from the oven and let it rest for a few minutes.

8. Garnish the Lemon Herb Baked Tilapia with chopped fresh parsley before serving.

9. Serve the baked tilapia hot with your favorite side dishes, such as steamed vegetables, rice, or salad.

10. Enjoy the light and refreshing flavors of this Lemon Herb Baked Tilapia!

72. Mango and Black Bean Quinoa Salad

Ingredients:
- 1 cup quinoa, rinsed
- 2 cups water or vegetable broth
- 1 ripe mango, peeled, pitted, and diced
- 1 cup cooked black beans (canned beans, rinsed and drained, can be used)
- 1 red bell pepper, diced
- 1/4 cup red onion, finely chopped
- 1/4 cup fresh cilantro, chopped
- Juice of 2 limes
- 2 tablespoons extra virgin olive oil
- 1 tablespoon honey or maple syrup
- 1 teaspoon ground cumin
- Salt and pepper to taste
- Optional: sliced avocado for serving

Instructions:
1. In a medium saucepan, combine the quinoa and water or vegetable broth. Bring to a boil, then reduce the heat to low, cover, and simmer for about 15 minutes, or until the quinoa is cooked and the liquid is absorbed. Remove from heat and let it cool slightly.

2. In a large mixing bowl, combine the cooked quinoa, diced mango, cooked black beans, diced red bell pepper, finely chopped red onion, and chopped fresh cilantro.

3. In a small bowl, whisk together the lime juice, extra virgin olive oil, honey or maple syrup, ground cumin, salt, and pepper to make the dressing.

4. Pour the dressing over the quinoa salad and toss until everything is evenly coated.

5. Taste and adjust the seasoning if necessary.

6. If desired, add sliced avocado to the salad for extra creaminess and flavor.

7. Serve the Mango and Black Bean Quinoa Salad chilled or at room temperature as a refreshing side dish or light meal.

8. Enjoy the vibrant colors and delicious flavors of this nutritious salad!

Feel free to customize the salad by adding other ingredients such as diced cucumber, cherry tomatoes, or jalapeño for some heat.

73. Coconut Curry Vegetables

Ingredients:
- 2 tablespoons coconut oil
- 1 onion, diced
- 3 cloves garlic, minced
- 1 tablespoon grated ginger
- 2 tablespoons curry powder
- 1 teaspoon ground turmeric
- 1 teaspoon ground cumin
- 1/2 teaspoon ground coriander
- 1/4 teaspoon cayenne pepper (optional, for heat)
- 1 can (14 oz/400ml) coconut milk
- 2 cups mixed vegetables (such as bell peppers, carrots, broccoli, cauliflower, snap peas, etc.), chopped
- Salt and pepper to taste
- Fresh cilantro, chopped, for garnish (optional)
- Cooked rice or naan bread, for serving

Instructions:

1. Heat the coconut oil in a large skillet or saucepan over medium heat.

2. Add the diced onion to the skillet and cook until softened, about 3-4 minutes.

3. Stir in the minced garlic and grated ginger, and cook for another 1-2 minutes until fragrant.

4. Add the curry powder, ground turmeric, ground cumin, ground coriander, and cayenne pepper (if using) to the skillet. Cook, stirring constantly, for about 1 minute to toast the spices and release their flavors.

5. Pour in the coconut milk and stir until the spices are well combined with the coconut milk.

6. Add the chopped mixed vegetables to the skillet and stir to coat them evenly with the coconut curry sauce.

7. Cover the skillet and simmer the vegetables in the coconut curry sauce for about 10-15 minutes, or until they are tender but still crisp.

8. Taste and adjust the seasoning with salt and pepper as needed. Once the vegetables are cooked to your liking, remove the skillet from the heat.

9. Serve the Coconut Curry Vegetables hot over cooked rice or with naan bread. Garnish with chopped fresh cilantro if desired.

10. Enjoy the rich and aromatic flavors of this Coconut Curry Vegetables dish as a satisfying and comforting meal!

Feel free to customize the recipe by adding your favorite vegetables or protein sources such as tofu, chickpeas, or shrimp. Adjust the spice level according to your preference by adding more or less cayenne pepper.

74. Quinoa Stuffed Bell Peppers

Ingredients:
- 4 large bell peppers
- 1 cup quinoa
- 2 cups vegetable broth or water
- 1 tbsp olive oil
- 1 onion, diced
- 2 cloves garlic, minced
- 1 carrot, diced
- 1 zucchini, diced
- 1 cup cherry tomatoes, halved
- 1 cup cooked black beans
- 1 tsp ground cumin
- 1 tsp paprika
- Salt and pepper to taste
- 1 cup shredded cheese
- Fresh parsley or cilantro for garnish (optional)

Instructions:
1. Halve and deseed bell peppers, set aside.

2. Cook quinoa in broth, set aside.

3. Sauté onion, garlic, carrot, zucchini, tomatoes, beans, cumin, paprika, salt, and pepper.

4. Mix cooked quinoa and veggies, add half the cheese.

5. Stuff bell peppers, bake covered at 375°F for 25-30 mins.

6. Top with remaining cheese, bake uncovered for 5-10 mins.

7. Garnish and serve.

75. Grilled Chicken Caesar Salad (using a light dressing)

Ingredients:
- 2 boneless, skinless chicken breasts
- 1 head romaine lettuce, chopped
- 1/4 cup grated Parmesan cheese
- 1/4 cup croutons (optional)
- Olive oil for grilling
- Salt and pepper to taste

For the dressing:
- 1/4 cup plain Greek yogurt
- 1 tablespoon olive oil
- 1 tablespoon lemon juice
- 1 clove garlic, minced
- 1 teaspoon Dijon mustard
- Salt and pepper to taste

Instructions:
1. Preheat your grill to medium-high heat.

2. Season the chicken breasts with salt and pepper. Drizzle with olive oil.

3. Grill the chicken breasts for about 6-7 minutes per side, or until cooked through and no longer pink in the center. Remove from the grill and let them rest for a few minutes before slicing.

4. While the chicken is grilling, prepare the dressing. In a small bowl, whisk together the Greek yogurt, olive oil, lemon juice, minced garlic, Dijon mustard, salt, and pepper until smooth and well combined. Adjust seasoning to taste.

5. In a large salad bowl, toss the chopped romaine lettuce with the grated Parmesan cheese.

6. Slice the grilled chicken breasts and add them to the salad.

7. Drizzle the dressing over the salad and toss until everything is evenly coated.

8. If using, sprinkle croutons over the top of the salad for added crunch.

9. Serve the Grilled Chicken Caesar Salad immediately as a satisfying and nutritious meal.

10. Enjoy the delicious flavors of this lighter version of the classic Caesar salad!

76. Ratatouille Stuffed Peppers

Ingredients:
- 4 bell peppers, any color
- 1 small eggplant, diced
- 1 zucchini, diced
- 1 yellow squash, diced
- 1 onion, diced
- 2 cloves garlic, minced
- 1 can (14 oz) diced tomatoes
- 2 tablespoons tomato paste
- 1 teaspoon dried thyme
- 1 teaspoon dried oregano
- Salt and pepper to taste
- Olive oil for cooking
- Grated Parmesan cheese for topping (optional)
- Fresh basil leaves for garnish (optional)

Instructions:
1. Preheat your oven to 375°F (190°C).

2. Cut the tops off the bell peppers and remove the seeds and membranes. Place the hollowed-out peppers in a baking dish and set aside.

3. Heat some olive oil in a large skillet over medium heat. Add the diced eggplant, zucchini, yellow squash, onion, and minced garlic. Cook, stirring occasionally, until the vegetables are tender, about 8-10 minutes.

4. Stir in the diced tomatoes, tomato paste, dried thyme, dried oregano, salt, and pepper. Cook for another 5 minutes to allow the flavors to meld together.

5. Spoon the ratatouille mixture into the hollowed-out bell peppers, pressing down gently to pack it in.

6. Cover the baking dish with aluminum foil and bake in the preheated oven for 25-30 minutes, or until the peppers are tender.

7. If using, sprinkle grated Parmesan cheese over the top of each stuffed pepper during the last 5 minutes of baking.

8. Once done, remove the stuffed peppers from the oven and let them cool slightly before serving.

9. Garnish with fresh basil leaves if desired. Serve the Ratatouille Stuffed Peppers hot as a flavorful and satisfying vegetarian meal. Enjoy the delicious combination of flavors and textures in these stuffed peppers!

Feel free to customize the recipe by adding other vegetables such as mushrooms or carrots, or by incorporating cooked grains like quinoa or rice into the filling.

77. Avocado and Black Bean Quesadillas

Ingredients:
- 4 large flour tortillas
- 1 ripe avocado, peeled, pitted, and sliced
- 1 can (15 oz) black beans, drained and rinsed
- 1 cup shredded cheese (such as cheddar or Monterey Jack)
- 1/2 cup salsa
- 2 green onions, chopped
- 1/4 cup chopped fresh cilantro (optional)
- Olive oil or cooking spray

Instructions:
1. Heat a large skillet or griddle over medium heat.

2. Lay one tortilla flat on a clean surface. Arrange avocado slices evenly over half of the tortilla.

3. Spoon black beans over the avocado slices.

4. Sprinkle shredded cheese over the beans.

5. Drizzle salsa over the cheese.

6. Sprinkle chopped green onions and cilantro (if using) over the top.

7. Fold the tortilla in half over the filling to create a half-moon shape.

8. Lightly brush the outside of the quesadilla with olive oil or coat the skillet with cooking spray.

9. Place the quesadilla in the skillet and cook for 2-3 minutes on each side, or until golden brown and crispy, and the cheese is melted.

10. Repeat the process with the remaining tortillas and filling ingredients.

11. Once done, remove the quesadillas from the skillet and let them cool for a minute.

12. Cut each quesadilla into wedges and serve hot.

13. Enjoy your Avocado and Black Bean Quesadillas with additional salsa, guacamole, or sour cream on the side if desired.

78. Lemon Garlic Roasted Brussels Sprouts

Ingredients:
- 1 lb Brussels sprouts, trimmed and halved
- 2 tablespoons olive oil
- 3 cloves garlic, minced
- Zest of 1 lemon
- Juice of 1/2 lemon
- Salt and pepper to taste
- Optional: grated Parmesan cheese for serving

Instructions:
1. Preheat your oven to 400°F (200°C). Line a baking sheet with parchment paper or foil.

2. In a large bowl, toss the Brussels sprouts with olive oil, minced garlic, lemon zest, lemon juice, salt, and pepper until evenly coated.

3. Spread the Brussels sprouts in a single layer on the prepared baking sheet.

4. Roast in the preheated oven for 20-25 minutes, or until the Brussels sprouts are tender and caramelized, stirring halfway through to ensure even cooking.

5. Once done, remove the Brussels sprouts from the oven and transfer them to a serving dish.

6. If desired, sprinkle grated Parmesan cheese over the roasted Brussels sprouts before serving.

7. Serve hot as a flavorful side dish or appetizer.

8. Enjoy the delicious combination of lemon and garlic flavors in these roasted Brussels sprouts!

Feel free to adjust the seasoning according to your taste preferences and add additional herbs or spices for extra flavor.

79. Greek Quinoa Stuffed Tomatoes

Ingredients:

- 4 large tomatoes
- 1 cup quinoa, rinsed
- 2 cups vegetable broth or water
- 1 tablespoon olive oil
- 1 small onion, finely chopped
- 2 cloves garlic, minced
- 1/2 cup chopped cucumber
- 1/2 cup chopped bell pepper (any color)
- 1/4 cup chopped Kalamata olives
- 1/4 cup crumbled feta cheese
- 2 tablespoons chopped fresh parsley
- 1 tablespoon chopped fresh dill
- Juice of 1 lemon
- Salt and pepper to taste

Instructions:

1. Preheat your oven to 375°F (190°C).

2. Slice off the tops of the tomatoes and scoop out the seeds and pulp with a spoon. Place the hollowed-out tomatoes in a baking dish and set aside.

3. In a medium saucepan, bring the vegetable broth or water to a boil. Add the quinoa, reduce the heat to low, cover, and simmer for about 15 minutes, or until the quinoa is cooked and the liquid is absorbed. Remove from heat and let it cool slightly.

4. In a large skillet, heat the olive oil over medium heat. Add the chopped onion and minced garlic, and sauté until softened and fragrant, about 3-4 minutes.

5. Add the cooked quinoa to the skillet with the onion and garlic. Stir in the chopped cucumber, chopped bell pepper, chopped Kalamata olives, crumbled feta cheese, chopped fresh parsley, chopped fresh dill, and lemon juice. Season with salt and pepper to taste. Stir until well combined.

6. Spoon the quinoa mixture into the hollowed-out tomatoes, pressing down gently to pack it in.

7. Place the stuffed tomatoes in the preheated oven and bake for about 20-25 minutes, or until the tomatoes are tender and the filling is heated through.

8. Once done, remove the stuffed tomatoes from the oven and let them cool slightly before serving.

9. Serve the Greek Quinoa Stuffed Tomatoes warm as a flavorful and nutritious main dish or side. Enjoy the delicious Mediterranean flavors of these stuffed tomatoes!

80. Walnut Crusted Baked Salmon

Ingredients:
- 4 salmon fillets (about 6 oz each), skin removed
- 1 cup walnuts, finely chopped
- 2 tablespoons Dijon mustard
- 1 tablespoon honey or maple syrup
- 1 tablespoon lemon juice
- 1 teaspoon dried thyme
- Salt and pepper to taste
- Lemon wedges for serving
- Fresh parsley, chopped, for garnish (optional)

Instructions:
1. Preheat your oven to 400°F (200°C). Line a baking sheet with parchment paper or foil for easy cleanup.

2. In a small bowl, mix together the chopped walnuts, Dijon mustard, honey or maple syrup, lemon juice, dried thyme, salt, and pepper to create the walnut crust.

3. Pat the salmon fillets dry with paper towels and place them on the prepared baking sheet.

4. Divide the walnut crust mixture evenly among the salmon fillets, pressing it gently onto the top of each fillet to form a coating.

5. Bake the walnut crusted salmon in the preheated oven for about 12-15 minutes, or until the salmon is cooked through and flakes easily with a fork.

6. Once done, remove the salmon from the oven and let it rest for a few minutes.

7. Serve the Walnut Crusted Baked Salmon hot, garnished with lemon wedges and chopped fresh parsley if desired.

8. Enjoy the delicious combination of flavors and textures in this simple and elegant dish!

Feel free to adjust the seasoning and sweetness level of the walnut crust according to your taste preferences. You can also add a sprinkle of lemon zest or chopped fresh herbs to enhance the flavor further.

• Types of Inflammatory Arthritis

Inflammatory arthritis encompasses several types of arthritis characterized by inflammation of the joints. Here are some of the main types:

1. Rheumatoid Arthritis (RA): RA is an autoimmune disorder where the immune system mistakenly attacks the synovium (the lining of the membranes that surround the joints), leading to inflammation, pain, swelling, and eventually joint damage and deformity.

2. Psoriatic Arthritis (PsA): PsA is a type of arthritis that affects some individuals with psoriasis, a chronic skin condition characterized by patches of red, inflamed skin. It causes joint pain, stiffness, and swelling, often affecting the fingers, toes, lower back, and other joints.

3. Ankylosing Spondylitis (AS): AS primarily affects the spine and sacroiliac joints (the joints that connect the base of the spine to the pelvis). It causes inflammation of the spinal joints, leading to pain and stiffness, which can result in a hunched-forward posture.

4. Reactive Arthritis: Reactive arthritis typically develops in response to an infection in another part of the body, such as the intestines or urinary tract. It commonly affects the joints, causing pain, swelling, and stiffness.

5. Juvenile Idiopathic Arthritis (JIA): JIA refers to a group of chronic arthritis conditions that affect children and adolescents under the age of 16. The exact cause is unknown, but it involves inflammation of the joints, leading to pain, stiffness, and potential joint damage.

6. Systemic Lupus Erythematosus (SLE): Lupus is a chronic autoimmune disease that can affect various parts of the body, including the joints. Inflammation caused by lupus can lead to arthritis symptoms, such as joint pain and swelling.

These are just a few examples of inflammatory arthritis types, and there are other less common types as well. Each type has its own specific symptoms, diagnostic criteria, and treatment approaches. It's important for individuals experiencing symptoms of arthritis to consult with a healthcare professional for proper diagnosis and management.

• How Diet Influences Inflammation

Diet plays a significant role in inflammation, and certain dietary choices can either promote or reduce inflammation in the body. Here's how diet influences inflammation:

1. Anti-inflammatory Foods: Incorporating foods that have anti-inflammatory properties can help reduce inflammation in the body. These include:

- Fatty fish rich in omega-3 fatty acids, such as salmon, mackerel, and sardines.

- Fruits and vegetables high in antioxidants, vitamins, and minerals, such as berries, cherries, leafy greens, and cruciferous vegetables like broccoli and Brussels sprouts.

- Healthy fats, such as those found in olive oil, avocados, and nuts.

- Whole grains, like brown rice, quinoa, and whole wheat, which are rich in fiber and nutrients.

2. Pro-inflammatory Foods: On the other hand, certain foods can promote inflammation in the body when consumed in excess. These include:

- Processed and refined carbohydrates, such as white bread, pastries, and sugary snacks, which can spike blood sugar levels and promote inflammation.

- Trans fats and saturated fats found in fried foods, processed snacks, and fatty meats, which can trigger inflammation and contribute to chronic diseases.

- Excessive intake of omega-6 fatty acids, often found in refined vegetable oils like soybean oil and corn oil, which can imbalance the omega-3 to omega-6 ratio and promote inflammation.

3. Gut Health: The health of the gut microbiota also influences inflammation. Consuming a diet high in fiber from fruits, vegetables, and whole grains can promote a healthy balance of gut bacteria, which in turn can reduce inflammation. Fermented foods like yogurt, kefir, and sauerkraut can also support gut health.

4. Individual Sensitivities: Certain individuals may have specific food sensitivities or intolerances that can trigger inflammation. Common culprits include gluten, dairy, and nightshade vegetables like tomatoes and peppers. Identifying and eliminating these trigger foods can help reduce inflammation in susceptible individuals.

5. Overall Diet Quality: In general, following a balanced and varied diet rich in whole, nutrient-dense foods while minimizing processed and unhealthy options can help maintain a healthy inflammatory response in the body.

• Key Anti-Inflammatory Nutrients

Several nutrients have been shown to have anti-inflammatory properties and can play a crucial role in reducing inflammation in the body. Here are some key anti-inflammatory nutrients:

1. Omega-3 Fatty Acids: Omega-3 fatty acids, particularly EPA (eicosapentaenoic acid) and DHA (docosahexaenoic acid), found in fatty fish like salmon, mackerel, and sardines, as well as in flaxseeds, chia seeds, and walnuts, have potent anti-inflammatory effects. They help reduce the production of pro-inflammatory substances in the body and promote the synthesis of anti-inflammatory molecules.

2. Polyphenols: Polyphenols are plant compounds found in fruits, vegetables, herbs, spices, tea, and red wine. They have antioxidant and anti-inflammatory properties and can help combat inflammation. Examples of polyphenol-rich foods include berries, cherries, grapes, citrus fruits, green tea, and dark chocolate.

3. Vitamin C: Vitamin C is a powerful antioxidant that can help reduce inflammation by scavenging free radicals and inhibiting the production of inflammatory cytokines. Foods rich in vitamin C include citrus fruits, strawberries, kiwi, bell peppers, broccoli, and kale.

4. Vitamin E: Vitamin E is another antioxidant that can help protect cells from inflammation-induced damage. It works synergistically with vitamin C to neutralize free radicals. Good food sources of vitamin E include nuts, seeds, vegetable oils, spinach, and avocados.

5. Curcumin: Curcumin is the active compound found in turmeric, a spice commonly used in Indian cuisine. It has potent anti-inflammatory properties and has been shown to inhibit inflammation pathways in the body. Incorporating turmeric into your diet or taking curcumin supplements can help reduce inflammation.

6. Quercetin: Quercetin is a flavonoid found in various fruits, vegetables, and herbs. It possesses anti-inflammatory and antioxidant properties and can help reduce inflammation by inhibiting inflammatory enzymes and signaling pathways. Foods rich in quercetin include apples, onions, berries, kale, and broccoli.

7. Magnesium: Magnesium is a mineral involved in over 300 enzymatic reactions in the body, including those related to inflammation. It can help modulate inflammatory processes and reduce systemic inflammation. Good food sources of magnesium include leafy green vegetables, nuts, seeds, whole grains, and legumes.

Incorporating these key nutrients into your diet through a variety of whole, nutrient-dense foods can help support your body's natural anti-inflammatory mechanisms and promote overall health and well-being.

• Top Anti-Inflammatory Foods

1. *Fatty Fish:* Fatty fish such as salmon, mackerel, sardines, and trout are rich in omega-3 fatty acids, particularly EPA and DHA, which have potent anti-inflammatory properties.

2. *Berries:* Berries like strawberries, blueberries, raspberries, and blackberries are packed with antioxidants and flavonoids, which help combat inflammation and oxidative stress.

3. *Leafy Greens:* Leafy green vegetables like spinach, kale, Swiss chard, and collard greens are excellent sources of vitamins, minerals, and phytonutrients that have anti-inflammatory effects.

4. *Nuts and Seeds:* Nuts such as almonds, walnuts, and Brazil nuts, as well as seeds like flaxseeds, chia seeds, and hemp seeds, are rich in healthy fats, fiber, and antioxidants that can help reduce inflammation.

5. *Turmeric:* Turmeric contains curcumin, a compound with powerful anti-inflammatory and antioxidant properties. Incorporating turmeric into your cooking or consuming turmeric supplements can help alleviate inflammation.

6. *Ginger:* Ginger is another spice with potent anti-inflammatory properties. It contains gingerol, which has been shown to reduce inflammation and alleviate symptoms of inflammatory conditions like osteoarthritis.

7. *Cherries:* Cherries, especially tart cherries, are rich in anthocyanins and other antioxidants that have anti-inflammatory effects. Consuming cherries or cherry juice may help reduce inflammation and alleviate symptoms of gout and arthritis.

8. *Olive Oil:* Extra virgin olive oil is rich in monounsaturated fats and contains oleocanthal, a compound with anti-inflammatory properties similar to ibuprofen. It is a cornerstone of the Mediterranean diet, which is known for its anti-inflammatory effects.

9. *Cruciferous Vegetables:* Vegetables like broccoli, cauliflower, Brussels sprouts, and cabbage are members of the cruciferous family and contain sulforaphane, a compound with anti-inflammatory and cancer-fighting properties.

10. *Tomatoes:* Tomatoes are rich in lycopene, a powerful antioxidant that helps reduce inflammation and protect against chronic diseases like cardiovascular disease and certain cancers.

Incorporating these top anti-inflammatory foods into your diet can help support your body's natural defense against inflammation and promote overall health and well-being.

• Foods to Avoid

1. *Processed and Refined Carbohydrates:* Foods made with refined grains, such as white bread, white rice, pasta, pastries, and sugary snacks, can spike blood sugar levels and promote inflammation. Opt for whole grains instead.

2. *Sugary Beverages:* Soft drinks, fruit juices, energy drinks, and other sugary beverages are high in added sugars, which can promote inflammation and contribute to chronic diseases like obesity, type 2 diabetes, and heart disease.

3. *Trans Fats*: Trans fats are found in partially hydrogenated oils used in fried foods, baked goods, margarine, and processed snacks. They can trigger inflammation and increase the risk of heart disease and other health problems. Read labels and avoid products containing trans fats.

4. *Saturated Fats:* Foods high in saturated fats, such as fatty cuts of meat, full-fat dairy products, butter, and cheese, can promote inflammation and increase levels of LDL cholesterol (the "bad" cholesterol). Choose lean protein sources and opt for low-fat or plant-based alternatives.

5. *Processed and Fried Foods:* Processed foods like chips, crackers, frozen meals, and fast food often contain unhealthy fats, added sugars, and artificial additives that can promote inflammation. Fried foods are also high in unhealthy fats and should be limited.

6. *Excessive Alcohol:* While moderate alcohol consumption may have some health benefits, excessive alcohol intake can promote inflammation and damage organs like the liver. Limit alcohol consumption to moderate levels, if at all.

7. *Highly Processed Foods:* Highly processed foods like packaged snacks, convenience meals, and fast food often contain unhealthy fats, sugars, and additives that can contribute to inflammation. Choose whole, minimally processed foods whenever possible.

8. *Artificial Sweeteners:* Some studies suggest that artificial sweeteners like aspartame, saccharin, and sucralose may disrupt gut microbiota and promote inflammation. Limit consumption of foods and beverages containing artificial sweeteners.

9. *Refined Vegetable Oils:* Refined vegetable oils like soybean oil, corn oil, and sunflower oil are high in omega-6 fatty acids, which, when consumed in excess, can promote inflammation. Opt for healthier fats like olive oil, avocado oil, and coconut oil.

10. *Highly Allergenic Foods:* Certain individuals may be sensitive or allergic to specific foods, such as gluten, dairy, eggs, and nightshade vegetables like tomatoes, peppers, and eggplants. Pay attention to how your body reacts to these foods and limit or avoid them if necessary

Meal Planning for Arthritis

Meal planning for arthritis involves choosing foods that can help reduce inflammation, support joint health, and manage symptoms associated with arthritis. Here's a basic guide for meal planning for arthritis:

1. Include Anti-Inflammatory Foods: Base your meals around anti-inflammatory foods like fatty fish (salmon, mackerel), leafy greens (spinach, kale), berries (blueberries, strawberries), nuts and seeds (walnuts, flaxseeds), olive oil, turmeric, and ginger.

2.Emphasize Omega-3 Fatty Acids: Incorporate omega-3 rich foods into your diet regularly. Include fatty fish in your meals at least twice a week. You can also add flaxseeds, chia seeds, hemp seeds, and walnuts to salads, yogurt, smoothies, or oatmeal.

3. Load Up on Fruits and Vegetables: Aim to include a variety of colorful fruits and vegetables in your meals and snacks. These are rich in antioxidants, vitamins, and minerals that help reduce inflammation and support overall health. Try to have at least one serving of vegetables with every meal.

4. Choose Whole Grains: Opt for whole grains like brown rice, quinoa, barley, oats, and whole wheat bread instead of refined grains. Whole grains provide fiber, vitamins, and minerals, which can help maintain a healthy weight and reduce inflammation.

5. Incorporate Lean Protein: Include lean protein sources such as skinless poultry, lean cuts of meat, tofu, tempeh, legumes (beans, lentils), and low-fat dairy products. Protein is essential for muscle strength and repair, which can help support joint health.

6. Healthy Fats: Include sources of healthy fats in your diet, such as olive oil, avocado, nuts, and seeds. These fats have anti-inflammatory properties and can help reduce inflammation in the body.

7. Limit Processed Foods: Minimize the intake of processed and packaged foods, which often contain unhealthy fats, added sugars, and preservatives that can contribute to inflammation. Instead, focus on whole, minimally processed foods.

8. Stay Hydrated: Drink plenty of water throughout the day to stay hydrated. Herbal teas, coconut water, and infused water with fruits and herbs are also good options. Limit sugary beverages and excessive caffeine intake, as they can contribute to inflammation.

9. Manage Portions: Pay attention to portion sizes to maintain a healthy weight, as excess weight can put added stress on your joints. Use smaller plates, bowls, and utensils to help control portion sizes.

10. Consult with a Registered Dietitian: Consider working with a registered dietitian who can help you create a personalized meal plan tailored to your nutritional needs, preferences, and health goals.

• **Sample Meal Plans**

Here are two sample meal plans for a day, focusing on anti-inflammatory foods and suitable for individuals with arthritis:

Sample Meal Plan 1:
Breakfast:
- Greek yogurt parfait with mixed berries (blueberries, strawberries, raspberries), topped with a sprinkle of ground flaxseeds and a drizzle of honey.

- Whole grain toast with mashed avocado and sliced tomatoes.

- Green tea or herbal tea.

Lunch:
- Grilled salmon salad with mixed greens (spinach, arugula, kale), cherry tomatoes, cucumber slices, and sliced avocado.

- Quinoa salad with roasted vegetables (bell peppers, zucchini, eggplant) and a lemon-tahini dressing.

- Fresh fruit salad for dessert (pineapple, mango, kiwi).

Snack:
- Carrot and celery sticks with hummus.

- Handful of mixed nuts (almonds, walnuts, pistachios).

Dinner:
- Baked chicken breast seasoned with turmeric and served with steamed broccoli and brown rice.

- Mixed green salad with olive oil and balsamic vinegar dressing.

- Steamed edamame beans as a side dish.

- Herbal tea or water with lemon.

Sample Meal Plan 2:
Breakfast:
- Oatmeal topped with sliced banana, chopped walnuts, and a drizzle of honey.

- Smoothie made with spinach, frozen berries, almond milk, and a scoop of protein powder.

- Green tea or herbal tea.

Lunch:
- Lentil soup with carrots, celery, onions, and spinach.

- Whole grain pita bread with hummus and sliced cucumbers.

- Mixed berry salad with spinach, walnuts, and a light vinaigrette dressing.

- Orange slices for dessert.

Snack:
- Apple slices with almond butter.

- Low-fat Greek yogurt with a sprinkle of cinnamon.

Dinner:
- Grilled tofu stir-fry with bell peppers, broccoli, snap peas, and mushrooms, served with brown rice.

- Side salad with mixed greens, cherry tomatoes, and avocado, dressed with olive oil and lemon juice.

- Steamed asparagus spears.

- Herbal tea or water with lime.

These sample meal plans provide a variety of nutrient-dense foods rich in anti-inflammatory compounds to help manage symptoms of arthritis and promote overall health and well-being. Adjust portion sizes and ingredients based on individual preferences and dietary restrictions.

Tips for Meal Prep and Grocery Shopping

Meal Prep:

1. Plan Ahead: Take some time to plan your meals for the week, considering your schedule and dietary preferences. Choose recipes that are simple to prepare and can be easily modified to accommodate any physical limitations you may have.

2. Use Adaptive Tools: Consider using adaptive kitchen tools and gadgets to make meal prep easier, such as jar openers, easy-grip utensils, and electric kitchen appliances like food processors and slow cookers.

3. Prep in Stages: Break down meal prep tasks into smaller, manageable steps, and spread them out over the course of a few days if needed. For example, chop vegetables one day, cook grains and proteins another day, and assemble meals the day before or the morning of.

4. Batch Cooking: Cook large batches of staple foods like grains, proteins, and sauces that can be used in multiple meals throughout the week. Store leftovers in portioned containers for easy reheating and serving.

5. Prep Convenience Foods: Purchase pre-cut vegetables, pre-cooked grains, and canned beans or lentils to save time and effort in the kitchen. Just be mindful of added sodium and preservatives in packaged foods.

6. Freeze Individual Portions: If you have limited mobility or energy, consider freezing individual portions of meals for quick and easy reheating when you don't feel up to cooking.

Grocery Shopping:

1. Make a List: Before heading to the grocery store, make a list of the items you need based on your meal plan. Organize your list by categories (e.g., produce, dairy, pantry staples) to streamline your shopping trip.

2. Shop Online: Consider using online grocery shopping and delivery services, which can save you time and energy, especially if mobility is an issue. Many grocery stores and retailers offer this service for a small fee or even free with a minimum purchase.

3. Choose Convenient Options: Look for pre-cut fruits and vegetables, pre-washed salad greens, and pre-cooked proteins like rotisserie chicken to minimize prep time and effort.

4. Shop the Perimeter: Focus on shopping the perimeter of the grocery store, where you'll find fresh produce, lean proteins, dairy products, and whole grains. Try to avoid the inner aisles, where processed and packaged foods are typically located.

5. Read Labels: When selecting packaged foods, read the nutrition labels carefully to check for added sugars, unhealthy fats, and high sodium content. Choose products with minimal ingredients and avoid those with long lists of additives and preservatives.

6. Stock Up on Staples: Keep your pantry stocked with staple items like whole grains, canned beans, herbs and spices, healthy oils, and low-sodium broths or sauces, so you always have the basics on hand to whip up a nutritious meal.

By incorporating these tips into your meal prep and grocery shopping routine, you can make the process more manageable and enjoyable, even with arthritis. Don't hesitate to ask for assistance from family members, friends, or caregivers if needed, and remember to listen to your body and prioritize self-care throughout the process.

Creating Balanced Meals

1. *Include a Protein Source:* Protein is essential for building and repairing tissues, supporting immune function, and maintaining muscle mass. Choose lean protein sources such as poultry, fish, tofu, beans, lentils, eggs, or dairy products. Aim to include a palm-sized portion of protein in each meal.

2. *Add Colorful Vegetables:* Vegetables are rich in vitamins, minerals, fiber, and antioxidants that are essential for good health. Aim to fill half of your plate with a variety of colorful vegetables such as leafy greens, peppers, carrots, broccoli, and tomatoes. Choose a mix of raw and cooked vegetables for optimal nutrient intake.

3. *Incorporate Whole Grains:* Whole grains provide complex carbohydrates, fiber, vitamins, and minerals that help keep you feeling full and satisfied. Choose whole grains such as brown rice, quinoa, barley, oats, whole wheat bread, or whole grain pasta. Aim to make at least half of your grain choices whole grains.

4. *Include Healthy Fats:* Healthy fats are important for brain health, hormone production, and nutrient absorption. Incorporate sources of healthy fats such as avocados, nuts, seeds, olive oil, fatty fish (salmon, mackerel, sardines), and nut butters. Be mindful of portion sizes, as fats are calorie-dense.

5. *Don't Forget about Fruit:* Fruit provides natural sweetness, vitamins, minerals, and fiber. Include a serving of fruit with your meals or as a snack. Choose whole fruits like berries, apples, oranges, bananas, or grapes, and limit fruit juices and dried fruits, which can be higher in sugar and calories.

6. *Watch Portion Sizes:* Pay attention to portion sizes to avoid overeating. Use visual cues like your hand or common household items to estimate appropriate portion sizes. Aim for a balanced plate with protein, vegetables, and grains, and be mindful of high-calorie condiments and sauces.

7. *Stay Hydrated:* Drink plenty of water throughout the day to stay hydrated. Aim for at least eight glasses of water per day, or more if you're physically active or live in a hot climate. Limit sugary beverages and alcohol, which can add empty calories and contribute to dehydration.

8. *Balance Your Plate:* Aim to create meals that include a balance of protein, carbohydrates, and fats. Choose a variety of foods from each food group to ensure you're getting a wide range of nutrients. Experiment with different flavors, textures, and cooking methods to keep meals interesting and satisfying.

As we reach the end of **"Healing Recipes and Anti-Inflammatory Tips"**, we hope that you have found inspiration, knowledge, and practical tools to help manage your arthritis through the power of nutrition. Our journey together through these pages has been about more than just recipes; it's been about embracing a lifestyle that supports your overall well-being.

Living with arthritis can be challenging, but the right diet can make a significant difference. By incorporating the anti-inflammatory foods and recipes from this book into your daily routine, you are taking proactive steps towards reducing inflammation, alleviating pain, and enhancing your quality of life.

Remember, the journey to better health is a marathon, not a sprint. Small, consistent changes often lead to the most significant improvements over time. Be patient with yourself and celebrate each positive step you take. Listen to your body, adjust your diet as needed, and don't hesitate to consult with healthcare professionals for personalized advice.

In addition to following the recipes and tips provided, we encourage you to continue exploring new ingredients and cooking methods that align with an anti-inflammatory diet. Make this lifestyle your own, tailoring it to fit your tastes and preferences. Experiment with flavors, try new dishes, and most importantly, enjoy the process.

We hope that the meals you prepare from this book bring comfort and satisfaction to your life. Cooking and eating should be pleasurable activities, even when following dietary guidelines for health reasons. Our aim has been to make this journey as delicious and enjoyable as possible.

Thank you for allowing us to be part of your path to better health. We wish you success, joy, and vitality as you continue to explore the healing potential of food. May your kitchen be filled with vibrant, nourishing meals that support your journey to wellness.

Warm regards,

Gustav Henning

9 798326 056368